# RENAL DIET COOKBOOK

Easy Recipes for Healthy Kidneys and to Manage Ibs Symptoms

(Essential Recipes Specially Designed to Treat Kidney Diseases)

**Robert Sweet**

Published by Alex Howard

# © Robert Sweet

All Rights Reserved

*Renal Diet Cookbook: Easy Recipes for Healthy Kidneys and to Manage Ibs Symptoms (Essential Recipes Specially Designed to Treat Kidney Diseases)*

**ISBN 978-1-989891-86-5**

**Legal & Disclaimer**

The information contained in this book is not designed to replace or take the place of any form of medicine or professional medical advice. The information in this book has been provided for educational and entertainment purposes only.

# Table of contents

# Part 1

# Introduction

We have combined all of the recipes in these two books to provide you with plenty of inspiration and meals to keep you going for weeks and months. Going through kidney disease can be hard enough at the best of times, without having to stress about the foods you're eating and the meals to cook. These recipes have been created with renal-friendly ingredients to help bring enjoyment to cooking as well as eating again. There are plenty of breakfasts, entrées, desserts and drinks to choose from, and if you're lifestyle is a little hectic try any one of the 50+ slow cooker recipes included. Each recipe is listed with important nutritional information, helping you to plan out your meals according to your specific needs.

As well as the recipes, we've included an overview of kidney disease and its different stages as well as the possible causes and potential symptoms you may be experiencing. The shopping and food lists aim to help you stock up your kitchen with essential items, furthermore we hope that the eating out and travelling advice will provide you with the confidence you need to continue socialising and doing the things you love again whilst experiencing the earlier stages of the disease.

Whether you or someone you know has been diagnosed, you think you may be suffering from the symptoms but are not sure, or if you have a family history of chronic kidney disease and want to find out more about it, the good news is that with the right diet, medication and lifestyle, it is possible to delay and even prevent the need for dialysis and kidney transplants. It is always absolutely vital that you use this information alongside professional guidance; make sure you see your doctor if you are experiencing, or suspect you may be experiencing, kidney disease. It's also essential you continue to see your doctor, nutritionist or nephrologist regularly after your diagnosis and consult them before you make any dietary or lifestyle changes.

We wish you all the best in the kitchen and in health!

# C1: the truth about kidney disease

Our kidneys perform vital functions in our body to help keep us healthy; they help to maintain mineral levels such as potassium, sodium and phosphorous, as well as regulate water levels. The kidneys also remove waste and extra fluids from our body after digestion, muscle activity or from exposure to certain medications and chemicals.

The enzyme renin, secreted by the kidneys, helps to regulate blood pressure and create erythropoietin, the hormone that helps trigger the formation of red blood cells by bone marrow. These are both vital for healthy functioning. Last but not least, our kidneys generate an active vitamin D that we need for healthy bones.

If left untreated, kidney disease could lead to kidney failure. Treatment for kidney failure is usually dialysis or a kidney transplant. However, kidney disease can be slowed down and treated with the right balance of medication, nutrition and advice from your professional consultant.

If you experience kidney disease for longer than three months and it goes untreated then you will develop chronic kidney disease. Often, the symptoms of kidney disease can go unnoticed and therefore this can be dangerous as some patients develop chronic kidney disease without even being aware that they have experienced the earlier stages.

## Causes of Kidney Disease

High blood pressure and diabetes (both type 1 and type 2) are the top two causes of kidney disease. However, if you do have diabetes, this can be controlled by monitoring blood sugar levels in order to help to prevent kidney disease as well as coronary heart disease and strokes.

Other causes include:

Immune system diseases such as lupus, hepatitis B and C, and HIV,

Frequent urinary tract infections affecting your kidneys (pyelonephritis) could cause scars to build up which can lead to damage of the kidneys,

Inflammation of the glomeruli (the tiny filters inside the kidneys) can occur after strep infections,

An inherited kidney disease called polycystic kidney disease causes fluid filled cysts to form in the kidneys,

NSAIDS drugs such as naproxen and ibuprofen used for a prolonged period of time can permanently damage the kidneys,

Taking illegal drugs such as heroin,

Long-term exposure to certain chemicals can cause the breakdown of kidney functions.

# Acute Renal Failure

If you experience a sudden, total loss of kidney function, this is known as acute renal failure. There are three top causes of renal failure:

Lack of blood reaching the kidneys,

Urine not being expelled from the kidneys,

Direct damage to the kidneys.

There are several factors that can cause these three things to happen including:

Traumatic injuries causing severe blood loss,

Sepsis (an infection that can cause the body to go into shock),

Severe dehydration (particularly in athletes because of the sudden breakdown of muscles and the release of large amounts of a protein called myoglobin that causes harm to the kidneys),

An enlarged prostate,

Drug/toxins,

Eclampsia/pre-eclampsia/HELLP Syndrome in pregnant women.

# Symptoms of Kidney Disease

There are many different symptoms that you may experience with kidney disease and these include:

• Fatigue,

• Loss of appetite,

• Difficulty concentrating,

• Sleep problems,

• Needing to urinate more frequently,

• Blood in urine,

- Foamy urine,

- Muscle cramps or twitches,

- Swelling in the ankles or feet (edema),

- Dry or itchy skin,

- Puffiness around your eyes.

Experiencing one or more of these symptoms may be an indication that you have kidney disease and you should consult a professional if you do experience any of the above. As these symptoms may also be a result of another illness or disease, kidney disease can often go unnoticed. It is even more important you ask your doctor about kidney disease if you do suffer from diabetes, high blood pressure, if you have a family history of kidney disease, or are over 60 years old.

Symptoms of acute renal failure include:

- Shortness of breath due to fluid build up,

- Reduced amount of urine,

- Ongoing nausea,

- Weakness,

- A pain or intense pressure on your chest.

Remember the only way of knowing you have kidney disease at any stage is through consulting a professional who will conduct a urinalysis, measure urine volume, take blood samples or use ultrasound to diagnose you. It is vital once you have been diagnosed that you follow the professional advice given to you, in order to prevent kidney failure. This will usually involve a combination of medication; a healthy lifestyle; a reduction of over-the-counter medications such as aspirin; as well as toxins in the home such as tobacco and cleaning products.

# Five Stages of Kidney Disease

The different stages of kidney disease are determined by the Glomerular Filtration Rate (GFR). This is the process where the kidneys filter the blood that removes fluids and wastes. The GFR calculation determines how well the blood is being filtered.

The GFR is calculated using a formula that includes your age, race, gender, and serum creatinine levels. The lower the number, the further along your kidney disease will be. As always, this would have to be monitored and diagnosed by a professional.

**Stage 1 kidney disease: GFR = approximately 90+**

At this stage, you may not have any symptoms and so this is why it is often unnoticed. If your doctor does determine you have Stage 1 chronic kidney disease (CKD) it will usually be due to diabetes or high blood pressure. If there is a family history of polycystic kidney disease, you have a greater chance of experiencing chronic kidney disease. Therefore it is wise to go for check ups in order to ensure you do not have kidney disease, especially if you also suffer from any of the symptoms in the previous section.

Treatments: if diagnosed at this stage your doctor or nephrologist will recommend suitable treatment including medication and a healthy diet and lifestyle. The goal is to keep the kidneys functioning healthily on their own for as long as possible and to potentially avoid having to go through dialysis or a kidney transplant.

**Stage 2 kidney disease: GFR = 60-89**

Symptoms in stage 2 might include higher levels of urea or creatinine in your blood; there may be protein or blood in your urine.

Treatment as above for stage 1 kidney disease.

**Stage 3 kidney disease: 3a GFR = 45-59**

**3b GFR = 30-44**

This stage is classed as moderate kidney damage. Waste products will start to collect in the blood, which can cause uremia as the kidney function declines. This makes it more likely for you to develop kidney disease complications such as bone disease, anaemia, red blood cell shortage, or high blood pressure.

At this stage you may start to experience kidney pain in your lower back as well as sleep problems due to cramps in your legs. Fatigue is more common at this stage, along with swelling of extremities or edema, shortness of breath, and fluid retention. You might notice changes in your urine such as a foamy consistency or changes in color to red, tea-colored, dark orange, or brown. Urination frequency may change.

Treatments: As Stage 3 kidney disease progresses it is recommended that you see a nephrologist who will perform a number of tests on your kidneys; you may also be sent to a dietician to help with your nutrition and meal plans.

If you have high blood pressure, your doctor will likely prescribe medicine.

ACE inhibitors and angiotensin receptor blockers have shown the potential to slow down kidney disease progression in people who don't suffer from high blood pressure. You should ask your doctor about your medications and take them only as prescribed. You need to make sure you are taking your medicines, eating healthily, not smoking and exercising regularly to help prolong your kidney function. Talk with your doctor about an exercise plan; your doctor can also help you stop smoking. Kidney disease can't be cured but by following your doctor's advice and guidance you can slow down its progress.

**Stage 4 kidney disease: GFR = 15-30**

At this stage, waste collects in the blood causing uremia as kidney function decreases. Complications such as high blood pressure, cardiovascular disease, heart disease, anaemia, and bone disease are likely to develop.

Treatments:

Appointments with your nephrologist are essential at least once every three months. They will conduct tests for creatinine, calcium, phosphorus, and haemoglobin levels to ascertain how well the kidneys are functioning. They will also monitor your blood pressure and diabetes if applicable. The ultimate goal is to keep your kidneys functioning for as long as possible but it is also possible that they may start to prepare your body for dialysis.

There are two main forms of dialysis:

Hemodialysis can be conducted either at a centre or in your home by a care partner. The dialysis machine will remove some of your blood through an artificial kidney or dialyzer to clean out the toxins that your kidneys can't remove by themselves any more. The cleaned blood is then returned to your body.

Peritoneal dialysis is needle free and you don't need anyone to assist you.

The last option would be to have a kidney transplant.

**Stage 5 kidney disease: GFR = 15 or below**

This is end stage kidney disease. The kidneys will have lost all function and will not be able to work effectively. You will need a kidney transplant or dialysis to survive.

With stage 5 kidney disease you might experience increased skin pigmentation; tingling of your hands or feet; muscle cramps; swelling around your eyes or ankles; little or no urine flow; unexplained itching; problems concentrating; and fatigue.

You may well start feeling better once you begin dialysis. By removing the toxins from the blood and replacing the functions with medicine you could enjoy a fairly good quality of life.

If a kidney transplant is recommended or desired, your nephrologist will explain the process to you and get your name on a waiting list for a donated kidney or help you find a living donor.

# C2: renal diet and nutrition

How Can Diet Affect Symptoms of Kidney Disease?

Changing your diet and lifestyle can go a long way in helping to control your kidney disease and prevent the later stages of kidney disease. This chapter will explore the different food and nutrient groups that you should familiarise yourself with if you have kidney disease. Please always consult your doctor before making changes to your diet.

**Carbohydrates** - should make up the majority of your diet, as they're the primary source of energy for your body.

There are two types of carbohydrates: complex and simple. An example of a simple carbohydrate is fruit. Fruit is packed with the fiber, vitamins and energy that your body needs. Examples of complex carbohydrates are grains, breads, and vegetables. All these carbohydrates provide minerals and vitamins as well as energy and fiber. Carbohydrates also play a vital role in balancing blood-sugar levels.

**Protein** - repairs tissue and builds muscle. Your body also uses protein to build antibodies. These are your body's defence against disease. Animal foods are the primary sources of protein such as milk, beef, eggs, chicken and pork. Protein can also be found in some plants. Legumes, nuts, and soy bean products are all good sources of proteins. Vegetables also contain small amounts of protein. Protein is essential for good health however in later stages of chronic kidney disease your renal dietitian may have you cut back on protein intake to help reduce stress on the kidneys.

**Fats-** transport vitamins K, E, D, and A to your cells. They produce the hormones testosterone and estrogen. Some fats contain fatty acids that are good for your skin. These fatty acids also make up linings of cells in the body and help with the transmission of nerves. However, too much fat or the wrong kind of fat in your diet can cause weight gain, leading to heart disease and many other problems with your health.

There are two types of fats: unsaturated and saturated. Meat and dairy products are saturated fats. Too much of these fats can elevate your cholesterol; this cholesterol is what causes heart disease and clogged arteries. The food and drug administration recommend reducing your saturated fat intake. Nuts, fish, and certain oils are good sources of unsaturated fats and all help to reduce cholesterol. Trans fats will raise cholesterol levels just like saturated fats. The FDA suggests you choose food that is low in trans fats and saturated fats. Processed foods usually contain trans fats.

**Sodium, potassium, and phosphorus** - are the three main minerals balanced by the kidneys. As chronic kidney disease gets worse, some foods will need to be avoided as your kidneys will no longer be able to get rid of the excess from these minerals. Blood tests will be conducted to monitor the levels of these minerals.

**Sodium** -In the early stages of kidney disease, a low sodium diet may be all you need if you have high blood pressure. Your kidneys cannot get rid of excess fluid and sodium from your body whilst experiencing kidney disease. To help identify salt in foods look for ingredients on the label such as baking powder, sodium or brine. Generally, children and adults should eat less than 2,300 mg of sodium a day.

Kidney disease stage 1 and 2 = 1-3.5g per day

Kidney disease stage 3 - 4 = 1-2.5g per day

Kidney disease stage 5 = 1-2g per day

**Potassium** -Kidneys usually get rid of excess potassium in your urine to maintain normal levels in your blood. When experiencing kidney disease they can no longer do this effectively.

Hyperkalemia (or high potassium levels) occurs in the later stages of kidney disease. Symptoms of high potassium are a slow pulse, numbness, weakness, and nausea.

Kidney disease stage 1 and 2 = 2-5g per day

Kidney disease stage 3 - 4 =2-4g per day

Kidney disease stage 5 = 2-2.5per day

**Phosphorus** - Since your kidneys can no longer remove phosphorus from your blood and urine, hyperphosphatemia or high phosphorus may become a problem during stage 4 or 5 kidney disease.

Kidney disease stage 1 and 2 = up to 1000mg per day

Kidney disease stage 3 - 4 (GFR of 25-90+)= p to 1000mg per day

Kidney disease stage 4 (GFR of 15-25) = up to 750mgper day

Kidney disease stage 4 (GFR of 5-15) = up to 7mg per kg of body weight

(Capicchiano, 2017)

# C3 -renal diet and lifestyle guidance

**1. Always follow your dietician's advice in conjunction with any research or cookbooks you use:** During kidney disease this is extremely important. They can advise you about sodium, phosphorous and potassium content of favorite foods and give you recommendations on how to reduce your sodium intake. Your diet will be tailored to you, taking into account the stage of kidney disease you're in and any other illnesses or diseases you suffer from.

**2. Keep a Food Diary:** You should track what you're eating and drinking in order to stay within the guidelines and recommendations given to you. Apps such as My Fitness Pal make this extremely easy and even track many of the minerals and levels in foods including sodium, protein etc. There are also apps specifically made for kidney disease patients to track sodium, phosphorous and potassium levels.

**3. Read Food Labels:** Some foods have hidden sodium in them, even if they don't taste salty. You will need to cut back on the amount of canned, frozen, and processed foods you eat. Check your beverages for added sodium.

Check food labels to avoid: Potassium chloride, Tetrasodium phosphate, Sodium phosphate, Trisodium phosphate, Tricalcium phosphate, Phosphoric acid, Polyphosphate, Hexametaphosphate, Pyrophosphate, Monocalcium phosphate, Dicalcium phosphate, Aluminum phosphate, Sodium tripolyphosphate, Sodium polyphosphate.

**4. Flavor foods with fresh herbs and spices instead of shop-bought dressings and condiments:** These add flavor and variety to your meals and are not packed with sodium; spices also have many health benefits! Also stay away from salt substitutes and seasonings that contain potassium. Use citrus fruits and vinegars for dressings and to add flavor.

**5: Keep Up Your Appointments With Your Doctor or Nephrologist:**

13

Let your doctor know if you notice any swelling or changes in your weight.

**6. Monitor drink and fluid intake:** You have probably been told you need to drink up to eight glasses of water a day. This is true for a healthy body but for people experiencing the later stages of CKD, these fluids can build up and cause additional problems. The restriction of fluids will differ from person to person. Things to take into consideration are swelling, urine output, and weight gain. Your weight will be recorded before dialysis begins and once it's over. This is done to determine how much fluid to remove from your body. If you are undergoing haemodialysis, this will be recorded approximately three times a week. If you are undergoing peritoneal dialysis, your weight is recorded every day. If there is a significant weight gain you may be drinking too many fluids.

**7. Measure portion sizes** -Moderating your portion sizes is essential. Use smaller cups, bowls, or plates to avoid giving yourself oversized portions.

Measure your food so you can keep an accurate record of how much you are actually eating:

The size of your fist is equal to 1 cup.

The palm of your hand is equal to 3 ounces.

The tip of your thumb is equivalent to 1 teaspoon.

A poker chip is equal to 1 tablespoon.

Substitution Tips:

• Use plain white flour instead of whole-wheat/whole-grain

• Use all-purpose flour instead of self-raising,

• Use Stevia instead of sugar,

• Use egg whites rather than whole eggs,

- Use almond rice or soy milk instead of cows milk.

**8. Other Advice:** Be careful when eating in restaurants -ask for dressings and condiments on the side and watch out for soups and cured meats.

Watch out for convenience foods that are high in sodium.

Prepare your own meals and freeze them for later use.

Drain liquids from canned vegetables and fruits to help control potassium levels.

# Foods to Avoid:

- Cured meats
- Bacon and ham
- Cold cuts
- Frozen dinners
- Salted nuts
- Canned beans with salt added
- Canned entrées
- Raisins
- Oranges
- Cantaloupe
- Pumpkin
- Potatoes
- Dried beans
- Tomatoes
- Yogurt

- Ice Cream

- Milk

- Nuts and seeds

- Salt substitutes

- Molasses

- Chocolate

- Bottled coffee drinks

- Non-dairy creamers

- Cereal bars

- Enhanced chicken and meat

- Sodas

- Iced teas

- Flavored waters

- Sardines

- Offal

- Processed meats

- Dried beans

- Nuts and nut butters

- Avocado

- Pizza

- Biscuits, pancakes, waffles

- Corn tortillas

- Whole grain crackers, breads, cereals

- Bran

- Beer, chocolate drinks, cola, milk-based coffee

- Cheese

- Salted Butter

- Coconut

- Solid shortening

High potassium fruits should be avoided. A serving of the following listed fruits has more than 250 mg of potassium:

- 5 dried prunes or ½ cup prune juice

- 1/8 of a honeydew melon

- ¼ cup dates

- ½ cup orange juice or 1 small orange

- 1 small nectarine no bigger than 2 inches across

These vegetables have more than 250 mg of potassium in each 1.2 cup serving.

- Fresh beets

- Winter squash

- Tomatoes, juice, or ¼ cup sauce

- Sweet potatoes

- Potatoes

- Okra and Brussel sprouts

- ¼ avocado or 1 whole artichoke

# Foods To Enjoy:

**Red bell peppers** have low potassium but lots of flavor. They are also a good way to get folic acid, fiber, vitamin C, A, and B6. Red bell peppers also contain lycopene - an antioxidant that helps protect against cancer. A ½ cup serving contains 10 mg of phosphorus, 88 mg of potassium and 1 mg of sodium.

**Cabbage** contains phytochemicals - a chemical compound found in fruits and vegetables that helps break up free radicals. Phytochemicals are known to protect against cancer and help keep your heart healthy. Cabbage is high in vitamin C, K, B6, folic acid and fiber. A ½ cup serving contains just 9 mg of phosphorus, 60 mg potassium, and 6 mg sodium.

**Cauliflower** contains indoles, glucosinolates, and thiocyanates. These help the liver get rid of toxins that could damage cell membrane and DNA. A ½ cup serving of boiled cauliflower has 20 mg phosphorus, 88 mg potassium, 9 mg sodium.

Garlic helps reduce inflammation, keeps plaque from building on your teeth, and lowers cholesterol. Just one clove of garlic has 4 mg of phosphorus, 12 mg of potassium and 1 mg of sodium.

**Onion** contains quercetin an antioxidant that protects against cancers and helps heart disease. Onions contain chromium - a mineral that helps with protein, carbohydrate and fat metabolism. A ½ cup serving has 3 mg phosphorus, 116 mg potassium, and 3 mg sodium.

**Apples** prevent constipation, reduce cholesterol, reduce the risk of cancer, and protects against heart disease. Apples have anti-inflammatory compounds and are high in fiber. Just 1 medium apple with skin on has no sodium, 158 mg of potassium and 10 mg of phosphorus.

**Cranberries** can keep you from getting a bladder infection because they prevent bacteria from sticking to the bladder wall. Cranberries can also help the stomach from creating the bacteria that causes ulcers thus promoting good GI health. Cranberries can also protect against heart disease and cancer. A ½ cup cranberry juice cocktail has 3 mg phosphorus, 22 mg potassium, 3 mg sodium. A ¼ cup of cranberry sauce has 6 mg phosphorus, 17 mg potassium, and 35 mg sodium. A ½ cup of dried cranberries has 5 mg phosphorus, 24 mg potassium, and 2 mg sodium.

**Blueberries** help reduce inflammation. Blueberries contain manganese, fiber, and vitamin C. They also help protect the brain from the effects of aging. A ½ cup of fresh blueberries has 7 mg phosphorus, 65 mg potassium, and 4 mg sodium.

**Raspberries** contain phytonutrient ellagic acid which helps reduce free radical cell damage. They are high in vitamin C, manganese, folate, and fibre. A ½ cup of raspberries has 7 mg phosphorus, 93 mg potassium, 0 mg sodium.

**Strawberries** are a good source of manganese, vitamin C, and fibre. They provide anti-inflammatory and anti-cancer compounds and help to protect the heart. A ½ cup or 13 mg phosphorus, 120 mg potassium, 1 mg sodium.

**Cherries**, when eaten daily, can help reduce inflammation.. A ½ cup serving of fresh cherries has 15 mg phosphorus, 160 mg potassium, 0 mg sodium.

**Red grapes** protect against heart disease by reducing blood clots. They also help protect against inflammation and cancer. A ½ cup red grapes has 4 mg phosphorus, 88 mg potassium, 1 mg sodium.

**Egg whites** contain the highest quality protein and essential amino acids. 2 egg whites contain 10 mg phosphorus, 108 mg potassium, 110 mg sodium, and 7 grams protein.

**Fish** is a source of protein and anti-inflammatory fats known as omega-3s. Omega-3s help fight heart disease and cancer. It is recommended that you eat fish two times a week.

**Olive oil** helps fight against oxidation and inflammation. Virgin olive oils contain more antioxidants. 1 tablespoon olive oil serving contains less than 0 mg of phosphorus, less than a mg of potassium, and 1 mg of sodium.

**Vitamins and minerals**: Our bodies need vitamins to be able to function correctly. The best way to achieve this is make sure you eat a well-rounded diet. However, if you have chronic kidney disease, you may not be able to get all the recommended vitamins through diet alone. Vitamins that are usually recommended by your renal dietitian are vitamin C, biotin, pantothenic acid, niacin, vitamin B12, B6, B2, B1, and folic acid. You must consult your doctor or dietician before starting to take vitamin supplements.

# C4: eating out and shopping on a renal diet

## Advice for Dining Out

You don't have to miss out on your favorite restaurant or cuisines! Look out for small or half portions and ask your server for your foods to be cooked without extra salts, butters or sauces. Avoid fried foods and opt for grilled or poached instead.

If you know you are going out to eat, plan ahead. Look at the restaurant's menu beforehand and decide what you will order to avoid anxiety or stress on the night! Use the food lists above to help you choose and don't feel bad about asking them to cater for your needs. Be sure to take your phosphorus binders, if they have been prescribed to you. Take them with your meal instead of waiting until you get home.

# Advice for traveling

Whatever your travel plans, you will have to eat. If you plan ahead, you should be able to make a meal plan with your renal dietitian. Tell your dietitian where you are going and what you expect to eat at your destination.

Remember to pack any prescriptions you may have such as phosphate binders.

If you are diabetic remember to keep carbohydrate intake to a minimum. Try not to eat sweets such as sweetened drinks, fruit juices, cakes, pies, and candy. Don't consume salty foods like chips, crackers, and pretzels. Also limit condiments such as soy sauce, salad dressing, and ketchup. Keep a check on your blood sugar daily.

If going on a road trip or camping, avoid processed meats. If at all possible, use fresh-cooked meats, low-sodium deli meats, unsalted chicken or tuna.

Choose unsalted pretzels or crackers instead of potato chips. Salty foods need to be avoided if you are on a fluid restricted diet.

Take along nutritional drinks formulated for kidney patients. These can always be used as a meal replacement if need be.

Remember to check labels for sodium content.

Do not consume dairy products unless they are allowed as part of your diet plan.

1.      If you are going on a cruise, all those buffet foods are tempting to eat 24 hours a day. To help with this predicament try to select fruits, salads, and vegetables from the lists above.
2.      Remember to include a good source of protein with every meal and avoid breads and sauces that are salty. You could pack you own snacks to eat between meals.

3.     Let the cruise line know of your dietary needs, most are willing to prepare special foods for you. Low-sodium meal options may also be available.

4.     If you are going to be traveling abroad and don't speak the language, bring a phrasebook that has a section for ordering food.

## Cooking Tips

1. Grill, poach, roast or sauté meats instead of frying.

2. Steam or boil vegetables instead of frying.

3. Use healthy oils such as extra virgin olive oil to shallow fry.

4. Soak fruit and vegetables in warm water for 2 hours before cooking in order to reduce potassium levels – especially potatoes!

5. When using canned beans and vegetables, make sure to rinse and drain them.

6. Drain liquid from canned or frozen vegetables and fruits.

One Last Thing:

Always remember to use new recipes and ingredients after speaking to your doctor or dietician; your needs will be unique to you depending on the stage of Chronic Kidney Disease you're experiencing. We hope that with your doctor's advice, along with our guidance and recipes that you can continue to enjoy cooking, eating and sharing meal times with your love ones.

All the best and happy cooking!

# Breakfast

## Mediterranean Omelet
**SERVES 2 / PREP TIME: 2 MINUTES / COOK TIME: 10 MINUTES**

Fresh and healthy - packed with vitamins and protein.

1/2 red onion, peeled and thinly sliced
1 tbsp chopped chives

1 tbsp extra virgin olive oil
1 clove of garlic, crushed
2 eggs
Pinch of black pepper
1 tsp chopped parsley
1/4 cup almond milk

1.	Soak vegetables in water for up to 2 hours before cooking if possible.
2.	Beat eggs, pepper, herbs and almond milk in a separate bowl.
3.	Heat the oil in a skillet over a medium heat.
4.	Add the onion and garlic to the skillet and sauté on medium heat for a few minutes until soft.
5.	Pour the eggs evenly into the skillet and cook over a medium heat for 6-7minutes.
6.	Use a spatula to gently lift the edge; if it comes away easily, shake the pan a little.
7.	Flip or fold in half and continue to cook for a further 2-3 minutes.
8.	Sprinkle with the chives to serve.

**Per Serving:** Calories 186
Protein 7
Carbohydrates 7
Fat 7
Sodium 117
Potassium 124
Phosphorus 73

# Egg & Spinach Muffins
## SERVES 2 / PREP TIME: 10 MINUTES / COOK TIME: 25 MINUTES

So easy to prepare - just bung them in the oven!

1 4 hole muffin tin
1/3 cup green onions, washed diced

1 cup baby spinach leaves, washed

2 eggs

1 tsp sage, dried

1 tbsp almond milk

Pinch of black pepper

1.    Preheat oven to 180°C/350°F/Gas Mark 4.

2.    Line a 4 hole muffin tin with paper muffin wrappers.

3.    Layer each muffin case with 1/4 green onions and spinach.

4.    In a separate bowl, beat the eggs, sage, almond milk and black pepper.

5.    Pour 1/4 of the egg mixture into each muffin cup.

6.    Leave a little gap at the top of each case.

7.    Bake in the oven for 25 minutes, or until muffins have slightly risen and egg is cooked through.

8.    Remove muffins from pan and serve hot.

9.    Enjoy with a side salad if you wish.

**Per Serving:** Calories 92

Protein 7 g

Carbohydrates 2 g

Fat 0 g

Sodium 155 mg

Potassium 188 mg

Phosphorus 28 mg

# Lemon & Tarragon Crepes
## SERVES 2 / PREP TIME: 5 MINUTES / COOK TIME: 4 MINUTES

Light and bubbling with a hint of herbs and citrus to cut through!

2 eggs

1 tbsp tarragon, stalks removed and finely chopped

Pinch of black pepper

1-1/3 cups almond milk

3/4 cup all purpose white flour

1 tbsp coconut oil

1 lemon

1. Whisk eggs, tarragon, pepper and milk in a bowl.
2. Slowly sift in flour and whisk for 1 minute.
2. Heat a skillet over a medium to high heat.
3. Add coconut oil and allow to melt
4. Using a 1/4 cup measure, pour the batter evenly into the skillet.
5. Cook for 3-4 minutes until bubbling.
6. Loosen the edges of the crepe with a spatula and remove from the pan when golden on the bottom.
7. Repeat for the rest of the mixture.
8. Slice the lemon in half, squeeze over the crepes and serve.

**Per Serving:** Calories 408
Protein 15 g
Carbohydrates 60 g
Fat 10 g
Sodium 250 mg
Potassium 300 mg
Phosphorus 87 mg

# Parsley Omelet

**SERVES 2 / PREP TIME: 5 MINUTES / COOK TIME: 7 MINUTES**

A slight twist on the traditional omelet.

1 tbsp canola oil
1/4 onion, diced
1/4 fresh green bell pepper, diced
1 egg
2 egg whites
2 tbsp almond milk
2 sprigs fresh parsley

1. Heat the oil in a skillet over a medium heat.

2.      Add the diced onion and green pepper and sauté for 2 minutes.

3.      Whisk the eggs and almond milk together.

4.      Pour the eggs evenly across the vegetable mixture in the skillet.

5.      Allow to cook for 5-6 minutes on a medium heat until cooked through.

6.      Use your spatula to fold or flip and cook for a further minute.

7.      Sprinkle with parsley and cut in half to serve.

**Per Serving:** Calories 154

Protein 10 g

Carbohydrates 8 g

Fat 9 g

Sodium 47 mg

Potassium 307 mg

Phosphorus 76 mg

# Chili Scrambled Tortillas

## SERVES 2 / PREP TIME: 5 MINUTES / COOK TIME: 5 MINUTES

Kick-start your morning with these fiery wraps.

Non-stick cooking spray

2 egg whites

3 tbsp green chillies, diced

1/4 tsp ground cumin

1/2 tsp hot pepper sauce

2 flour tortillas

1.      Spray a skillet with non-stick cooking spray and heat over a medium heat.

2.      In a bowl, beat the egg whites with the green chillies, cumin and hot sauce.

3.      Pour egg mixture evenly into the skillet and cook for 1 to 2 minutes, stirring constantly until the eggs are cooked through.

4.      Heat tortillas for 20 seconds in a microwave or in a separate dry skillet over a medium heat.

5.      Top each tortilla with the scrambled eggs and roll.

6.      Enjoy warm!

**Per Serving:** Calories 247
Protein 12 g
Carbohydrates 36 g
Fat 3 g
Sodium 77 mg
Potassium 199 mg
Phosphorus 119 mg

# Speedy Beef & Bean Sprout Breaky
**SERVES 5 / PREP TIME: 2 MINUTES / COOK TIME: 25 MINUTES**

A protein and iron-rich breakfast which tastes delicious.

1 tbsp coconut oil for cooking
5 oz beef frying strips (organic grass-fed)
1/2 cup onions, finely diced
1 garlic clove, crushed
1 thumb-size piece of ginger, grated
1/2 cup bean sprouts
1 tbsp balsamic vinegar for dressing

1.      Heat 1/2 the coconut oil in a large skillet over a high heat.

2.      Add the beef frying strips and cook according to package directions.

3.      Remove beef from the skillet and place to one side.

4.      Add 1/2 coconut oil to the skillet and sauté the onions and garlic for 3-4 minutes over a medium heat until soft (don't brown!)

5.      Now add the ginger and bean sprouts.

6.	Serve 1/2 the vegetables on each serving dish and top with the beef strips.

7.	Drizzle with balsamic vinegar to serve.

**Per Serving:** Calories 69

Protein 12 g

Carbohydrates 3 g

Fat 1 g

Sodium 35 mg

Potassium 25 mg

Phosphorus 44 mg


# Chicken & Red Pepper Muffins
**SERVES 4 / PREP TIME: 10 MINUTES / COOK TIME: 30 MINUTES**

Savory breakfast muffins.


1 tbsp extra virgin olive oil

5 oz skinless chicken breasts, diced

1 red bell pepper, diced

1/2 cup spinach leaves, washed

2 English muffin

1 tbsp fresh basil, finely chopped (optional)

Pinch black pepper

1.	Heat 1/2 the olive oil in a skillet over a medium to high heat.

2.	Add the diced chicken and cook, turning occasionally for 20 minutes or according to package directions.

3.	Ensure the chicken is cooked through by sticking a sharp knife into the centre (it should come out clean).

4.	Remove from the pan and place to one side.

5.	Now add the red pepper to the skillet and sauté for 5-6 minutes or until soft.

6.	Add the spinach to the skillet and turn off the heat (the spinach will wilt slightly).

7.     Slice the English muffins in half and lightly toast in a toaster or under the grill.

8.     Meanwhile, mix the rest of the olive oil with the chopped basil and pepper.

9.     Top each half of the muffins with the chicken, followed by the vegetables and lastly drizzle with the basil oil.

**Per Serving:** Calories 139
Protein 10 g
Carbohydrates 14 g
Fat 6 g
Sodium 140 mg
Potassium 121 mg
Phosphorus 113 mg

# Vegetarian Eggs Benedict

**SERVES 4 / PREP TIME: 5 MINUTES / COOK TIME: 10 MINUTES**

Delicious healthy version of a posh brunch!

2 English muffins
1 tsp balsamic vinegar
3 cups water
4 eggs
1/2 cup spinach leaves

1.     Slice English muffins in half and toast them.

2.     Add the vinegar with one cup water into a large skillet.

3.     Bring to a boil and then lower the heat.

4.     Whilst stirring the water with a wooden spoon, crack the eggs into the water one at a time.

5.     Cover and simmer for 3 to 5 minutes or 1-2 minutes longer if you like hard yolks.

6.     Remove eggs with a slotted spoon and place on top of the English muffin halves; cover and keep warm.

7.     Top with freshly washed spinach leaves, a drizzle of balsamic vinegar, and a sprinkle of black pepper.

8.     Serve!

**Per Serving:** Calories 137

Protein 8 g

Carbohydrates 13 g

Fat 5 g

Sodium 176 mg

Potassium 174 mg

Phosphorus 126 mg

# Chili Tofu Scramble

## SERVES 2 / PREP TIME: 5 MINUTES / COOK TIME: 10 MINUTES

Tofu soaks up the flavors of whatever it's cooked with so add some spice!

1 tsp coconut oil

1/2 cup green onions, finely diced

1 red chilli, de-seeded and finely diced

6oz tofu, drained

1/2 lime

1. Heat the oil in a skillet or wok over a medium-high heat.

2. Add the green onions and sauté for 1-2 minutes.

3. Add the chili and sauté for 1 minute.

4. Add the tofu and cook for 5-6 minutes or according to package directions.

5. Slice the lime in half, squeeze over the tofu and stir.

6. Enjoy!

**Per Serving:** Calories 272

Protein 15 g

Carbohydrates 15 g

Fat 20 g

Sodium 15 mg

Potassium 289 mg

Phosphorus 113 mg

# Vanilla Pancakes

**SERVES 4 / PREP TIME: 5 MINUTES / COOK TIME: 5 MINUTES**

Sweet breakfast treat!

2/3 cup all-purpose flour
4 large eggs
1 cup unsweetened almond milk
1/4 tsp vanilla extract
Non-stick cooking spray

1.      Mix the flour with the sugar in a mixing bowl.
2.      Whisk the eggs into this mixture.
3.      Now add the milk and vanilla extract and beat until smooth.
4.      Heat a non-stick skillet over a medium heat with non-stick cooking spray.
5.      Pour 3 tablespoons of the batter into the skillet to cover.
6.      Cook for 1 minute until the pancake is brown on the bottom.
7.      Flip pancake and brown the other side.
8.      Remove and keep warm.
9.      Repeat until the batter is gone.
10.     Serve with your choice of topping.

**Per Serving:** Calories 102
Protein 7 g
Carbohydrates 3 g
Fat 5 g
Sodium 161 mg
Potassium 165 mg
Phosphorus 140 mg

# Renal-Friendly Rice Pudding

**SERVES 4 / PREP TIME: 5 MINUTES / COOK TIME: 25 MINUTES**

Wholesome and tasty!

2 cups water

2 cups rice milk

8 tbsp uncooked bulgur

1 cup canned apricots, drained

Pinch nutmeg

1.      Heat the water and milk in a pot over a medium-high heat.

2.      Bring to the boil and add the bulgur and apricots.

3.      Lower the heat to a simmer, stirring occasionally for 20-25 minutes.

4.      When the bulgur is soft, remove the pot from the heat and stir in the nutmeg.

5.      Leave to stand for 5 minutes.

6.      Stir through with a fork and serve.

**Per Serving:** Calories 119

Protein 5 g

Carbohydrates 26 g

Fat 1 g

Sodium 53 mg

Potassium 89 mg

Phosphorus 21 mg

# Apple & Cinnamon Muffins

## SERVES 6 / PREP TIME: 15 MINUTES / COOK TIME: 25 MINUTES

Treat yourself!

6 hole muffin tin

1 cup almond milk

1/2 tbsp apple cider vinegar

1 1/2 cups all-purpose flour

1/2 cup granulated sugar

1/4 tbsp baking soda (Ener-G substituate)

1/2 tsp ground cinnamon

1/4 cup canola oil

1 tbsp pure vanilla extract

1/2 cup apple sauce

1.      Preheat oven to 190°C/375°F/Gas Mark 5.
2.      Line the tin with paper cases.
3.      In a bowl, stir the almond milk and vinegar and leave to rest for 5 minutes.
4.      Meanwhile in a large bowl, mix the flour, sugar, baking soda substitute and cinnamon.
5.      Now add the oil and the vanilla to the milk mixture from earlier and stir through thoroughly.
6.      Now add the liquid mixture to the dry ingredients and stir until combined.
7.      Fold through the apple sauce.
8.      Spoon the mixture into the muffin cases and bake in the oven for 25 minutes or until golden and cooked through.
9.      Stick a knife into the centre and it should come out clean.
10.     Cool on a rack for 10 minutes before serving.

**Per Serving:** Calories 153
Protein 0 g
Carbohydrates 19 g
Fat 10 g
Sodium 270 mg
Potassium 72 mg
Phosphorus 47 mg

# Homemade Turkey Patties
## SERVES 4 / PREP TIME: 10 MINUTES / COOK TIME: 15 MINUTES

Patties are often unkind to our kidneys but these can be enjoyed guilt free!

1 tsp fennel seeds, crushed
6oz ground turkey
1/8 tsp garlic powder
1/8 tsp onion powder
1/4 tsp salt

1.      Crush the fennel seeds using a pestle and mortar or blender.

2.	In a bowl combine the turkey meat with the crushed fennel seeds, garlic powder, onion powder and salt (optional).

3.	Cover the bowl and refrigerate for as long as possible.

4.	Divide the turkey into 4 portions and flatten using the palms of your hands into patties to cook.

5.	Heat a non-stick skillet over a medium heat and add the patties until browned and cooked through (10-15 minutes).

**Per Serving:** Calories 69

Protein 7 g

Carbohydrates 1 g

Fat 3 g

Sodium 40 mg

Potassium 17 mg

Phosphorus 103 mg

# Breakfast Smoothie

**SERVES 4 / PREP TIME: 5 MINUTES / COOK TIME: NA**

Packed with Vitamin C - this sweet and sour combination tastes amazing.

1/2 grapefruit, peeled and diced

6 cups water

1/2 cup canned papaya, drained

1.	Add to a blender or smoothie maker and whiz up until smooth.

2.	Serve over ice.

**Per Serving:** Calories 18

Protein 4 g

Carbohydrates 15 g

Fat 20 g

Sodium 1 mg

Potassium 33 mg

Phosphorus 12 mg

# Smoked Salmon & Dill Bagels

**SERVES 2 / PREP TIME: 5 MINUTES / COOK TIME:NA**

Omega-3 and delicious-this is a great Sunday morning breakfast.

1 tbsp honey
1/2 lemon, juiced
1 tsp dill, fresh or dried
1 bagel
4oz smoked salmon
1.      Whisk the honey, lemon juice and dill together.
2.      Slice the bagel in half and lightly toast.
3.      Top with the salmon and squeeze the dressing over the top to serve.
**Per Serving:** Calories 215
Protein 15 g
Carbohydrates 30 g
Fat 3 g
Sodium 384 mg
Potassium 150 mg
Phosphorus 160 mg

# Winter Berry Smoothie

**SERVES 2 / PREP TIME: 5 MINUTES / COOK TIME: NA**

Vibrant in color and vitamins alike.

1/4 cup blackberries
1/4 cup cherries, pitted
1/4 cup cranberries
2 cups water
1.      Blend until smooth in a blender or smoothie maker.
2.      Serve right away.
**Per Serving:** Calories 21
Protein 2 g
Carbohydrates 5 g
Fat 0 g

Sodium 1 mg
Potassium 62 mg
Phosphorus 10 mg

# Breakfast in a Pan

## SERVES 4 / PREP TIME: 5 MINUTES / COOK TIME: 20 MINUTES

A One Pot Stop!

1 tbsp coconut oil
1 red bell pepper, diced
4 oz cooked skinless turkey breast
1/2 cup spinach leaves, washed
1 tsp oregano
1/4 cup scallions
2 egg whites

1.      Preheat the broiler to a medium-high heat.
2.      Into an oven proof skillet add the coconut oil over a medium heat until melted.
3.      Add the pepper and turkey and sauté for 10-15 minutes until soft.
4.      Now add the spinach, oregano and scallions and mix for 2 minutes.
5.      Add the egg whites and mix together.
6.      Place under the broiler for 4-5 minutes until the eggs are cooked.
7.      Divide into 2 portions and serve.

**Per Serving:** Calories 91
Protein 11 g
Carbohydrates 2 g
Fat 3 g
Sodium 37 mg
Potassium 113 mg
Phosphorus 80 mg

# Grilled Vegetables

**SERVES 4 / PREP TIME: 5 MINUTES / COOK TIME: 15 MINUTES**

Start your day with color!

1/4 green bell pepper, diced
1/4 red bell pepper, diced
1/4 yellow bell pepper, diced
1/4 zucchini,diced
1/4 red onion, diced
1 tbsp extra virgin olive oil
1 tsp thyme, fresh or dried
1 tsp oregano
1.      Preheat the broiler to a medium-high heat.
2.      Chop the vegetables into chunky pieces and if possible soak in warm water prior to use.
3.      Add the vegetables, oil and herbs to an oven dish and toss with your hands.
4.      Place under the broiler for 10-15 minutes or until vegetables are lightly grilled.
5.      Serve alone or with your choice of bread/salad.
**Per Serving:** Calories 43
Protein 0 g
Carbohydrates 2 g
Fat 3 g
Sodium 50 mg
Potassium 58 mg
Phosphorus 35 mg

# Kidney Friendly Porridge

**SERVES 2 / PREP TIME: 5 MINUTES / COOK TIME: 10 MINUTES**

Warm & sweet!

1 cup water

1/2 cup cream of wheat farina
1/2 cup canned pears, drained and sliced
Pinch ground nutmeg
1.      Bring the water to a boil in a saucepan.
2.      Remove from the heat and add the cream of wheat slowly.
3.      Stir continuously until combined.
4.      Return to the heat once more and bring to the boil.
5.      Lower the heat and cook for 3-4 minutes until thickened.
6.      Stir through the canned pears and nutmeg.
7.      Serve warm.
**Per Serving:** Calories 205
Protein 5 g
Carbohydrates 44 g
Fat 2 g
Sodium 3 mg
Potassium 92 mg
Phosphorus 18 mg

# Poultry

## Grilled Spiced Turkey
**SERVES 4 / PREP TIME: 5 MINUTES / COOK TIME: 20 MINUTES**

So simple and succulent.

1 tbsp olive oil
1 tsp cinnamon
1 tsp nutmeg
1 tsp curry powder
6oz turkey breast, skinless and sliced
1.      Whisk the oil and spices together and baste the turkey slices, coating thoroughly.
2.      Cover and leave to marinade for as long as possible (ideally overnight).

3.      When ready to cook, preheat the broiler to a medium-high heat and layer the turkey slices on a baking tray.
4.      Place under the broiler for 15-20 minutes or according to package directions.
5.      Turn occasionally.
**Per Serving:** Calories 101
Protein 9 g
Carbohydrates 6 g
Fat 11 g
Sodium 42 mg
Potassium 27 mg
Phosphorus 102 mg

# Herby Chicken Stew
## SERVES 6 / PREP TIME: 5 MINUTES / COOK TIME: 40 MINUTES
Warming and hearty!

1/2 cup eggplant, diced
1/2 red onion, diced
10 oz chicken breast, skinless and diced
1 tsp olive oil
Pinch of black pepper
1 cup water
1 tsp oregano, fresh or dried
1 tsp thyme, fresh or dried
1/2 cup white rice

1.      Soak vegetables in warm water prior to use if possible.
2.      Heat an oven-proof pot over a medium-high heat and add olive oil.
3.      Add the diced chicken breast and brown in the pot for 5-6 minutes, stirring to brown each side.
4.      Once the chicken is browned, lower the heat to medium and add the vegetables to the pot to sauté for 5-6 minutes - careful not to let vegetables brown.

5.     Add the water, herbs and pepper and bring to the boil.
6.     Reduce the heat and simmer (lid on) for 30-40 minutes or until chicken is thoroughly cooked through.
7.     Meanwhile, prepare your rice by rinsing in cold water first and then adding to a pan of cold water and bringing to the boil over a high heat.
8.     Reduce the heat to medium and cook for 15 minutes.
9.     Drain the rice and add back to the pan with the lid on to steam until the stew is ready.
10.    Serve the stew on a bed of rice and enjoy!
**Per Serving:** Calories 143
Protein 15 g
Carbohydrates 9 g
Fat 5 g
Sodium 12 mg
Potassium 20 mg
Phosphorus 153 mg

# Lemon & Herb Chicken Wraps
## SERVES 4 / PREP TIME: 5 MINUTES / COOK TIME: 30 MINUTES
Delicious for a quick snack!

1 tbsp olive oil
1 lemon
2 tbsp fresh cilantro, finely chopped
Pinch of black pepper
4 oz chicken breasts, skinless and sliced
1/2 red bell pepper, sliced
4 large iceberg lettuce leaves, washed
1.     Preheat the oven to 190°C/375°F/Gas Mark 5.
2.     Mix the oil, juice of 1/2 lemon, cilantro and black pepper.
3.     Marinate the chicken in the oil marinade, cover and leave in the fridge for as long as possible.
4.     Wrap the chicken in parchment paper, drizzling over the remaining marinade.

5.      Place in the oven in an oven dish for 25-30 minutes or until chicken is thoroughly cooked through and white inside.

6.      Divide the sliced bell pepper and layer onto each lettuce leaf.

7.      Divide the chicken onto each lettuce leaf and squeeze over the remaining lemon juice to taste.

8.      Season with a little extra black pepper if desired.

9.      Wrap and enjoy!

**Per Serving:** Calories 200

Protein 9 g

Carbohydrates 5 g

Fat 13 g

Sodium 25 mg

Potassium 125 mg

Phosphorus 81 mg

# Ginger & Bean Sprout Steak Stir-Fry
### SERVES 2 / PREP TIME: 4 MINUTES / COOK TIME: 10 MINUTES

Chinese inspired dish.

5oz lean organic beef steak, cut into strips

1 tsp coconut oil

1/4 cup bean sprouts

1 green onion, finely sliced

2 tsp fresh ginger, grated

1 garlic clove, minced

1 tsp nutmeg

1.      Slice the beef into strips and add to a dry hot pan, cooking for 4-5 minutes on each side or until they're cooked to your liking.

2.      Place to one side.

3.      Add the oil to a clean pan and sauté the bean sprouts and onions with the ginger, garlic and nutmeg for 1 minute.

4.      Serve the beef strips on a bed of the vegetables and enjoy.

**Per Serving:** Calories 227
Protein 13 g
Carbohydrates 13 g
Fat 23 g
Sodium 50 mg
Potassium 258 mg
Phosphorus 170 mg

# Carrot & Ginger Chicken Noodles
## SERVES 4 / PREP TIME: 5 MINUTES / COOK TIME: 10 MINUTES
Fresh and revitalising!

1 tsp coconut oil
4 oz chicken breasts, skinless and sliced
2 tsp fresh ginger, grated
1 garlic clove, minced
1 green onion, sliced
1 carrot, peeled and grated
1 lime
1 cup rice noodles, cooked

1.      Heat a wok or large pan over a medium-high heat.
2.      Add the coconut oil to a pan and once melted, add the sliced chicken and brown for 4-5 minutes.
3.      Now add the ginger and garlic and sauté for 4-5 minutes.
4.      Add the green onion, carrot and lime juice to the wok.
5.      Add the cooked noodles to the wok and toss until hot through.
6.      Serve piping hot and enjoy.

**Per Serving:** Calories 187
Protein 11 g
Carbohydrates 25 g
Fat 5 g
Sodium 39 mg
Potassium 91 mg
Phosphorus 178 mg

# Marjoram Chicken & Cauliflower Rice

**SERVES 4 / PREP TIME: 10 MINUTES / COOK TIME: 35 MINUTES**

An exciting take on your usual bland chicken meals.

1 cup cauliflower
1 tsp olive oil
1/2 onion, finely diced
2 tsp marjoram
6oz chicken breast, skinless and sliced
Pinch of black pepper

1.      Grate the cauliflower into rice-sized pieces (alternatively, use a food processor for 10 seconds to whiz up the cauliflower into small pieces).
2.      Heat the oil in a wok or pan over a medium heat.
3.      Sauté the onion in the wok for 4-5 minutes until it starts to soften.
4.      Sprinkle 1 tsp of the marjoram over the onions to coat.
5.      Add the chicken to the pan and sauté for 6-7 minutes to brown.
6.      Continue to cook on a medium heat for 20-25 minutes.
7.      Meanwhile, bring a pot of water to the boil over a high heat and add the cauliflower rice.
8.      Add 1 tsp marjoram to the pot.
9.      Turn down the heat immediately and cook the cauliflower for 5-6 minutes.
10.      Drain and add the cauliflower to the wok with the chicken.
11.      Stir and serve with a pinch of black pepper.

**Per Serving:** Calories 123
Protein 14 g
Carbohydrates 5 g
Fat 5 g
Sodium 17 mg
Potassium 125 mg
Phosphorus 125 mg

# Chicken & Water Chestnut Noodles
**SERVES 4 / PREP TIME: 5 MINUTES / COOK TIME: 25 MINUTES**

Delicious for lunch or dinner.

2 tsp coconut oil
4oz skinless chicken breasts, sliced
2 cup rice noodles
1 garlic clove, crushed
1 carrot, grated
1/2 cup water chestnuts, canned
1 lime, juiced

1. Heat 1 tsp oil on a medium heat in a skillet or wok.
2. Sauté the chicken breasts for about 15-20 minutes or until cooked through.
3. While cooking the chicken, place the noodles in a pot of boiling water for 5 minutes. Drain.
4. Add the garlic, carrot and water chestnuts to the wok and sauté for 3-4 minutes or until garlic aromas reach your nose!
5. Squeeze over the lime juice.
6. Serve hot straight away.

**Per Serving:** Calories 213
Protein 11 g
Carbohydrates 23 g
Fat 9 g
Sodium 27 mg
Potassium 4 mg
Phosphorus 99 mg

# Turkey Kebabs & Red Onion Salsa
**SERVES 8 / PREP TIME: 10 MINUTES /COOK TIME: 25 MINUTES**

A leaner meat teamed with a chili salsa.

**for the turkey:**
1/2 lemon, juiced
2 garlic cloves, minced

1 tsp cumin
1 tsp turmeric
8oz turkey breasts, cut into cubes
8 metal kebab skewers
Lemon wedges to garnish
**for the salsa:**
1 red onion, diced
1 lemon, juiced
1 tsp white wine vinegar
1 tsp black pepper
1 tbsp olive oil
1 tsp of chilli flakes
1.      Whisk the lemon juice, garlic, cumin and turmeric in a bowl to make your marinade.
2.      Skewer the turkey cubes using kebab sticks (metal).
3.      Baste the turkey on each side with the marinade, covering for as long as possible in the fridge or straight away if you're in a rush.
4.      When ready to cook, preheat the oven to 400°F/200 °C/Gas Mark 6 and bake for 20-25 minutes or until turkey is thoroughly cooked through.
5.      Prepare the salsa by mixing all the ingredients in a separate bowl.
6.      Serve the turkey kebabs, garnished with the lemon wedges and the salsa on the side.
**Per Serving:** Calories 67
Protein 9 g
Carbohydrates 2 g
Fat 2 g
Sodium 1 mg
Potassium 25 mg
Phosphorus 75 mg

# Griddled Chicken & Asparagus Linguine
## SERVES 4 / PREP TIME: 5 MINUTES / COOK TIME: 30 MINUTES

Light and fresh!

1 cup of asparagus stems
4oz skinless chicken breast, diced
1 tsp extra virgin olive oil
2 cups linguine pasta
1 tsp tarragon
Pinch of black pepper
1/2 lemon, juiced

1.   Prepare asparagus stems by removing the hard part at the base (about a cm).
2.   Heat a griddle pan on a medium to high heat and add the oil.
3.   Add the diced chicken and sauté for 15-20 minutes or until thoroughly cooked through.
4.   Meanwhile, cook your pasta in boiling water according to package directions.
5.   Place to one side.
6.   Wipe the pan clean and place over the heat again.
7.   Add the asparagus stems to the griddle pan for 5-10 minutes, turning to brown each side.
8.   Drain the pasta and add the chicken to the pasta, heating until piping hot throughout.
9.   Sprinkle with tarragon and black pepper and drizzle with a little lemon juice.
10.   Top each portion with the asparagus stems.
11.   Enjoy!

**Per Serving:** Calories 162
Protein 9 g
Carbohydrates 22 g
Fat 5 g
Sodium 85 mg
Potassium 67 mg
Phosphorus 134 mg

# Herby Breaded Chicken

**SERVES 4 / PREP TIME: 10 MINUTES / COOK TIME: 30 MINUTES**

Delicious!

2 pita bread
1/2 cup fresh basil
1 tsp extra virgin olive oil
2 egg whites
4oz chicken breasts, cut into strips
1 cup fresh watercress

1.      Preheat the oven to 350°f/170°c/Gas Mark 4.
2.      Add the pita bread, herbs and olive oil to a blender or pestle and mortar and blend into breadcrumbs.
3.      Pour into a shallow bowl.
4.      Whisk the egg whites in a separate shallow bowl.
5.      Individually, dip the chicken strips into the egg whites and then straight into the breadcrumbs to coat each side. (Add a little water to the breadcrumb mixture if you find it doesn't stick well).
6.      Place onto a baking sheet.
7.      Bake for at least 30 minutes in the oven, or until the chicken is completely cooked through.
8.      Serve the chicken with the watercress on the side.

**Per Serving:** Calories 151
Protein 12 g
Carbohydrates 18 g
Fat 5 g
Sodium 230 mg
Potassium 98 mg
Phosphorus 112 mg

# Chicken & White Wine Casserole

**SERVES 8 / PREP TIME: 10 MINUTES / COOK TIME: 40 MINUTES**

What a treat!

8oz skinless, boneless chicken breasts

1/2 cup all-purpose flour

2 1/2 tbsp unsalted butter

2 tbsp olive oil

1 medium onion, sliced

2 medium garlic cloves, sliced

1/2 cup dry white wine

3 tbsp fresh flat-leaf parsley, chopped

4 cups water

2 tbsp lemon juice

1.      Dice the chicken breasts.

2.      Add 1/2 cup flour and black pepper into a shallow dish.

3.      Dip the chicken into the first bowl of flour and shake to coat.

4.      Now, melt 1 tbsp of the butter in a large skillet over a medium-high heat.

5.      Add 1 tsp of the olive oil to the skillet.

6.      Add the floured chicken to the skillet and sauté for 10-15 minutes until browned.

7.      Add the onions and sauté for 3 minutes, whilst stirring.

8.      Add the garlic and sauté for 1 minute, whilst stirring.

9.      Add the wine to the skillet and turn up the heat to full.

10.     Bring to a boil and then turn down the heat and simmer until the liquid thickens, stirring occasionally.

11.     Add the reserved tsp flour to the water and stir.

12.     Now add this to the pan.

13.     Bring back to the boil on a high heat and then turn down to simmer for 10 minutes or until sauce is thickened.

14.     Ensure the chicken is thoroughly cooked through.

15.     Remove from the heat and stir in remaining 1-1/2 tablespoons butter and lemon juice.

16.     Serve right away with the chopped parsley to garnish.

**Per Serving:** Calories 108

Protein 5 g

Carbohydrates 2 g

Fat 7 g
Sodium 88 mg
Potassium 39 mg
Phosphorus 91 mg

# Filling Fajitas
**SERVES 4 / PREP TIME: 10 MINUTES / COOK TIME: 20 MINUTES**

A healthy version of the takeaway favorite.

4 Iceberg lettuce leaves
1 tsp olive oil
4 oz ground lean turkey
1/2 onion, finely diced
1 red bell pepper, finely diced
1 tsp paprika
1 tsp chili powder

1.    Carefully pull off the leaves from the lettuce and rinse.
2.    Mix the rest of the ingredients in a bowl.
3.    Heat the oil in a skillet over a medium to high heat.
4.    Add the turkey mixture to the pan and cook for 15-20 minutes or until cooked through.
5.    Once cooked, remove from the pan and add to the centre of each lettuce leaf before wrapping fajita style!
6.    Enjoy.

**Per Serving:** Calories 97
Protein 7 g
Carbohydrates 6 g
Fat 6 g
Sodium 83 mg
Potassium 139 mg
Phosphorus 82 mg

# Cranberry Chicken & Red Cabbage
**SERVES 4 / PREP TIME: 5 MINUTES / COOK TIME: 30 MINUTES**

This is a filling and healthy treat!

1/2 cup cranberries

1/4 cup brown sugar

1 tbsp apple cider vinegar

1 tsp cinnamon

1 cup water

1 tbsp olive oil

4oz boneless, skinless, chicken breasts

1/2 cup red onion, diced

1 cup of red cabbage, boiled

1. In a saucepan, add the cranberries, sugar, vinegar, cinnamon and 1 cup water over a medium-high heat.

2. Bring to the boil and allow to simmer until the sauce thickens for 15-20 minutes.

3. Meanwhile, heat the oil in a large skillet over a medium heat.

4. Add the chicken breasts and cook for 4-5 minutes on each side.

5. Add the onion and sauté until translucent. Take care not to let it brown.

6. Lower the heat, cover and cook for 15–20 minutes or until chicken breasts are thoroughly cooked through.

7. Add the boiled cabbage to the pan for 5 minutes or until warmed through.

8. Serve with the cranberry sauce.

**Per Serving:** Calories 180

Protein 5 g

Carbohydrates 32 g

Fat 4 g

Sodium 99 mg

Potassium 90 mg

Phosphorus 90 mg

# Caribbean Turkey

## SERVES 6 / PREP TIME: 5 MINUTES / COOK TIME: 40 MINUTES

Brings you the taste of the Caribbean!

1 garlic clove, minced
1 tbsp coconut oil, melted
2 tsp curry powder
1 tbsp Jamaican spice blend
6oz skinless turkey breast, diced
1 lime
1 cup brown rice

1.      Preheat the oven to 350°f/170°c/Gas Mark 4.
2.      Prepare the marinade by mixing garlic, coconut oil and spices together before pouring over the turkey.
3.      Add the turkey to a baking dish and place in the oven for 35-40 minutes.
4.      Meanwhile prepare your rice by bringing a pan of water to the boil.
5.      Add rice and cover and simmer for 20 minutes.
6.      Drain and cover the rice and return to the stove for 5 minutes.
7.      When the turkey is cooked through, serve on a bed of rice and squeeze fresh lime juice over the top.
8.      Enjoy.

**Per Serving:** Calories 149
Protein 10 g
Carbohydrates 16 g
Fat 3 g
Sodium 28 mg
Potassium 70 mg
Phosphorus 128 mg

# Turkey Chili and Brown Rice
**SERVES 6 / PREP TIME: 5 MINUTES / COOK TIME: 30 MINUTES**

Rustle this up in a flash and enjoy!

1 tbsp extra virgin olive oil
1 red onion, finely diced
1 garlic clove

1 red chili, finely diced

1 red bell pepper, finely diced

1 tsp curry powder

6oz lean ground turkey

1/4 cup water

2 cups brown rice

2 green onions, sliced

2 tbsp freshly chopped cilantro

1. Heat the oil in a skillet on a medium-high heat.

2. Throw in the onions and garlic and sauté for 5-6 minutes until translucent but take care not to brown.

3. Add the red pepper, chili and curry powder.

4. Now add the turkey mince and stir to combine.

5. Cook on a medium heat for 5 minutes or until turkey has browned.

6. Now add 1/4 cup water, cover the pan and leave to simmer on a low to medium heat for 20 minutes or until turkey is cooked through.

7. Meanwhile add your rice to a pan of cold water and bring to the boil.

8. Turn down the heat and simmer for 15 minutes.

9. Drain the rice, return the lid and steam for 5 minutes.

10. Serve the turkey chili on a bed of rice and garnish with freshly chopped cilantro and sliced green onions.

**Per Serving:** Calories 288

Protein 6 g

Carbohydrates 47 g

Fat 6 g

Sodium 38 mg

Potassium 69 mg

Phosphorus 126 mg

# Grilled Pineapple Chicken

**SERVES 4 / PREP TIME: 10 MINUTES / COOK TIME: 20 MINUTES**

Fruity and scrumptious.

1/2 iceberg lettuce or similar, washed and sliced

2 radishes, washed and sliced

1/2 cucumber, sliced

1 tsp extra virgin olive oil

1 tsp apple cider vinegar

4oz chicken breast, skinless

Pinch of black pepper

1 tsp dried thyme

1/2 cup canned pineapple rings, juices drained

1.      Preheat the broiler to a medium-high heat.

2.      Prepare your salad by combining lettuce, radish and cucumber. Cover and place in the fridge.

3.      Whisk oil and vinegar in a dressing bowl and place to one side.

4.      Preheat the broiler to a medium-high heat.

5.      Slice the chicken breast meat into strips.

6.      Place the chicken on a baking tray and sprinkle with black pepper and thyme.

7.      Place under the broiler for 10 minutes on each side or until thoroughly cooked through.

8.      Add the pineapple rings to the broiler 5 minutes before the chicken time is up.

9.      Serve the chicken strips and pineapple on a bed of salad and drizzle with the dressing prepared earlier.

**Per Serving:** Calories 87

Protein 26 g

Carbohydrates 6 g

Fat 4 g

Sodium 87 mg

Potassium 20 mg

Phosphorus 73 mg

# Lemon & Oregano Easy Cook Chicken
## SERVES 6 / PREP TIME: 10 MINUTES / COOK TIME: 25 MINUTES

A citrus twist on your usual chicken dish.

1/4 cup lemon juice

1/4 cup water

2 tbsp extra virgin olive oil

1 tsp dried oregano

1 bay leaf

6oz boneless, skinless chicken breasts, diced

1.      Combine lemon juice, chicken broth, olive oil, oregano and bay leaf in a glass dish or zip lock bag.

2.      Add chicken breasts, turn to coat, and marinate for at least 2 hours in the fridge.

3.      When ready to cook, preheat the broiler or grill to a medium-high heat.

4.      Broil or grill chicken on an oven dish for 10 minutes per side or until thoroughly cooked through - test with a sharp knife in the centre of the chicken breast to ensure that no liquid seeps out and the meat is white all the way through.

5.      Enjoy with your choice of rice, salad or pasta.

**Per Serving:** Calories 69

Protein 5 g

Carbohydrates 1 g

Fat 5 g

Sodium 87 mg

Potassium 14 mg

Phosphorus 75 mg

# Baked Turkey Breast & Eggplant

**SERVES 4 / PREP TIME: 10 MINUTES / COOK TIME: 40 MINUTES**

1 tbsp coconut oil

4oz boneless turkey breasts, sliced

1/2 eggplant, sliced into discs

2 tbsp olive oil

1/2 cup fresh cilantro, chopped

Pinch black pepper

1/4 cup low sodium chicken broth

1/4 cup arugula, washed

1. Preheat the oven to 350°f/170°c/Gas Mark 4.
2. Heat the coconut oil in a wok or skillet over a medium to high heat and sauté the sliced turkey breasts for 5 minutes or until browned.
3. Remove from the heat and place on a plate.
4. Layer a deep oven or lasagne dish with half the eggplant discs.
5. Drizzle over half the olive oil and half the herbs.
6. Layer half the turkey slices on the top and repeat with the rest of the eggplant, oil and herbs.
7. Sprinkle over black pepper.
8. Pour over the chicken broth and place in the oven for 20-30 minutes until turkey is completely cooked through and stock is bubbling.
9. Serve with a bed of arugula on the side.

**Per Serving:** Calories 138
Protein 9 g
Carbohydrates 0 g
Fat 11 g
Sodium 28 mg
Potassium 100 mg
Phosphorus 73 mg

# Festive Cranberry Turkey Breasts
## SERVES 4 / PREP TIME: 5 MINUTES / COOK TIME: 35 MINUTES

A Christmas treat that can be enjoyed all year round!

4oz turkey breasts
1 cup cranberries
1 tsp nutmeg
1 tsp cinnamon
1 tsp black pepper
1 cup water
1 tsp red wine vinegar
1. Preheat the broiler to a medium heat.

2.     Slice the turkey breast.

3.     Add to a lined baking tray and broil for 20-30 minutes or until cooked through.

4.     Meanwhile, heat a pot on a medium-high heat and add the rest of the ingredients.

5.     Allow to boil and then turn down the heat and simmer for 15 minutes or until reduced to a thick sauce.

6.     Serve the turkey breasts once cooked with a helping of cranberry sauce and your choice of vegetables.

**Per Serving:** Calories 63

Protein 9 g

Carbohydrates 4g

Fat 11 g

Sodium 28 mg

Potassium 101 mg

Phosphorus 72 mg

# Sweet and Sour Chicken

**SERVES 2 / PREP TIME: 10 MINUTES / COOK TIME: 30 MINUTES**

An oriental infused chicken dish.

1 tbsp coconut oil

6oz boneless, skinless chicken breasts, diced

1 cup celery, sliced

1 small onion, diced

1 green bell pepper, sliced

1 garlic clove, minced

1 cup reduced-sodium chicken broth

1/4 cup apple cider vinegar

1/2 cup canned pineapple chunks, juices drained

1 cup cooked rice

1.     Heat a wok or skillet over a medium-high heat and add coconut oil.

2.     Add the chicken, garlic, celery, pepper and onions and sauté for 5 minutes.

3.  Add the broth, vinegar and garlic.
4.  Cover and simmer over low heat for 15 minutes.
5.  Add the pineapple.
6.  Cook for a further 10 minutes, stirring occasionally.
7.  Ensure chicken is thoroughly cooked through.
8.  Serve over rice.

**Per Serving:** Calories 108
Protein 7 g
Carbohydrates 13 g
Fat 2 g
Sodium 105 mg
Potassium 140 mg
Phosphorus 126 mg

# Honey Mustard Grilled Chicken
## SERVES 2 / PREP TIME: 10 MINUTES / COOK TIME: 30 MINUTES

Honey and Mustard - mustard and honey can be beneficial to those with CKD in many ways but please as always consult your dietician before adding new ingredients.

1 tbsp deli-style mustard
1 tbsp honey
1 tsp apple cider vinegar
2 green onions, chopped
4oz boneless, skinless chicken breasts, sliced

1.  In a small bowl, combine the mustard, honey, vinegar and green onions to make a marinade and place to one side.
2.  Reserve 1/4 cup of the marinade to serve with the cooked chicken.
3.  Preheat the broiler or grill to a medium-high heat.
4.  Grill the chicken strips on an oven dish for 5 minutes.
5.  Brush with the marinade and turn several times until the chicken is thoroughly cooked through (approximately 15-20 minutes).

6.     Remove from the grill and serve with the rest of the honey-mustard sauce.

7.     Serve with a side of vegetables!

**Per Serving:** Calories 80

Protein 10 g

Carbohydrates 7 g

Fat 1 g

Sodium 172 mg

Potassium 25 mg

Phosphorus 156 mg

# MEAT

## Healthy Roast Dinner

**SERVES 4 / PREP TIME: MARINATE AS LONG AS POSSIBLE / COOK TIME: 45 MINUTES**

Rich in iron and B vitamins.

1 tbsp thyme

1 tsp pepper

1 tbsp olive oil

10 oz of lean rump steak

1 onion, peeled and sliced

4 turnips, peeled and diced

2 garlic cloves

1/4 cup fresh parsley, chopped

1.     Preheat the oven to 450°f/250°c/Gas Mark 8.

2.     Meanwhile, mix the thyme and black pepper with the olive oil.

3.     Coat the rump steak and allow to marinate for as long as possible.

4.     Add the rump steak to a shallow oven-proof dish and heat the hob to a high heat.

5. Sear each side of the beef steak for a few minutes until browned. If the baking dish is not suitable to place on the hob, do this in a separate skillet first.

6. Now add the vegetables and whole garlic cloves (skin on) to the baking dish (if your beef is already in the dish make sure you use tongs to lift it first).

7. Add the dish to the oven for 25 minutes before turning the heat down to 300°f/150°c/Gas Mark 2.

8. Continue to cook for a further 8 minutes and then remove and allow to rest (the beef will continue to cook in the resting time).

9. After 5 minutes, slice the steak with a carving knife and serve on top of the juicy vegetables. The garlic should be deliciously soft by now so serve this up too!

10. Garnish with fresh parsley.

**Per Serving:** Calories 183

Protein 20 g

Carbohydrates 6 g

Fat 8 g

Sodium 110 mg

Potassium 382 mg

Phosphorus 214 mg

# Mini Burgers

## SERVES 2 / PREP TIME: 5 MINUTES / COOK TIME: 20 MINUTES

Enjoy a treat now and then!

5 oz lean 100% grass-fed ground beef

1 tsp black pepper

1 tsp paprika

1 egg white

1 green onion, chopped

2 hamburger buns

1/4 cup arugula

1. Preheat the broiler/grill to a medium-high heat.

2.     Mix the ground beef with the herbs, egg white, spices and chopped green onion.

3.     Use your hands to form 2 patties (about 1 inch thick).

4.     Add to an oven proof baking tray and broil for 15 minutes or until meat is thoroughly cooked through. (Use a knife to insert into the centre - the juices should run clear).

5.     Slice your burger buns and stack with the burger and arugula.

**Per Serving:** Calories 227

Protein 17 g

Carbohydrates 23 g

Fat 7 g

Sodium 295 mg

Potassium 78 mg

Phosphorus 193 mg

# Slow-Cooked Beef Stew

## SERVES 4 / PREP TIME: 10 MINUTES / COOK TIME OVERNIGHT

Stick this in the slow cooker for succulent and tender meat.

1 tbsp of extra virgin olive oil

10 oz lean beef, cubed

1 onion, diced

1 red bell pepper, roughly chopped

4 cups of water

1 tsp cumin

1 tsp turmeric

1 tsp curry powder

1 tsp oregano

1 bay leaf

1/2 cauliflower, chopped and par-boiled

1.     Heat the olive oil in a skillet over a medium-high heat.

2.     Add the beef and cook for 5 minutes or until browned on each side.

3.    Add the onions, peppers and garlic to the slow cooker and pour in the water.
4.    Now add the herbs, spices and bay leaf.
5.    Then cover the slow cooker and cook for at least 8 hours or overnight.
6.    10 minutes before the end, add the cauliflower.
7.    Plate up and serve when ready to eat!
**Per Serving:** Calories 227
Protein 19 g
Carbohydrates 10 g
Fat 12 g
Sodium 72 mg
Potassium 313 mg
Phosphorus 193 mg

# Parsley Pork Meatballs
## SERVES 2 / PREP TIME: 5 MINUTES / COOK TIME: 30 MINUTES
Succulent pork meatballs with a garlic and olive oil sauce.

6 oz lean pork mince
2 tbsp extra virgin olive oil
1 garlic clove crushed
1/2 red onion, finely chopped
1 tsp dried sage
1 garlic clove, crushed
1/4 cup fresh parsley
1.    Mix the mince, 1 tbsp oil, 1 garlic clove, onion and sage in a bowl.
2.    Season with a little black pepper and separate into 8 balls, rolling with the palms of your hands.
3.    Heat 1 tbsp oil in a pan over a medium heat and add the meatballs for 5 minutes or until browned.
4.    Mix 1 tbsp olive oil, garlic and parsley in a separate bowl.
5.    Cover and lower heat to simmer for 15 minutes.
6.    Throw the parsley into the pan for the last minute.

7.      Serve Tapas style or with spaghetti for a bigger meal!
**Per Serving:** Calories 290

Protein 17 g

Carbohydrates 2 g

Fat 24 g

Sodium 5 mg

Potassium 53 mg

Phosphorus 44 mg

# Lime & Chili Beef Tortilla
**SERVES 2 / PREP TIME: 5 MINUTES / COOK TIME: 20 MINUTES**

Fresh and filling.

1 tsp olive oil

1 lime, juiced

1 tsp chili flakes

1 garlic clove, minced

1 tbsp coconut oil

5 oz lean beef mince

1/2 green bell pepper, sliced

1/4 cup green onions, chopped

1 tortilla

1.      Into a blender or pestle and mortar, add the olive oil, lime juice, chili flakes and garlic and blitz until nearly smooth.

1.      Heat the coconut oil in a skillet or wok over a medium-high heat.

2.      Add the beef mince and brown for 4 minutes.

3.      Now add the green pepper and continue to cook for a further 10 minutes.

4.      Add the green onions and marinade and mix through.

5.      Preheat the broiler or grill to a medium high heat.

6.      Slice the tortilla and place under the broiler until crispy.

7.      Serve the beef chilli with the tortilla chips on top.

8.      Enjoy!

**Per Serving:** Calories 243
Protein 18 g
Carbohydrates 16 g
Fat 12 g
Sodium 46 mg
Potassium 442 mg
Phosphorus 208 mg

# Nutmeg Pork Loin With White Cabbage
## SERVES 2 / PREP TIME: 5 MINUTES / COOK TIME: 20 MINUTES

Enjoy a taste of Germany!

2x 3oz lean pork loins
1 tsp nutmeg
A pinch black pepper
1 tbsp white wine vinegar
1/2 white cabbage, sliced
2 carrots, peeled and sliced
1.      Preheat the broiler to a medium-high heat.
2.      Sprinkle the pork with nutmeg on both sides.
3.      Add the pork loins to a baking tray and place under the broiler for 10-15 minutes or according to package guidelines.
4.      Meanwhile, place a pot of water over a medium-high heat.
5.      Add the pepper and vinegar to the pan.
6.      Now add the cabbage and carrots for 5-10 minutes or until soft.
7.      Drain the cabbage and carrots and serve with the pork.
8.      Enjoy!
**Per Serving:** Calories 97
Protein 13 g
Carbohydrates 7 g
Fat 2 g
Sodium 64 mg
Potassium 392 mg

Phosphorus 217 mg

# Beef & Eggplant Lasagna
## SERVES 4 / PREP TIME: 10 MINUTES / COOK TIME: 50 MINUTES

Creamy white sauce and succulent beef lasagna.

1 tsp olive oil
1 onion, diced
1 garlic clove, minced
12 oz lean ground beef
1 tsp cayenne pepper
1 tsp parsley
1 tsp black pepper
1/2 cup water
1 tbsp unsalted butter
1/4 cup plain flour
3/4 cup rice milk
1 tsp black pepper
1 eggplant, sliced vertically

1.      Preheat the oven to 350°f/170°c/Gas Mark 4.
2.      To prepare the beef: Heat the oil in a skillet on a medium -high heat and add the onions and garlic for 5 minutes until soft.
3.      Add the lean ground mince, season with herbs and spices, add water and cook for 10-15 minutes or until completely browned.
4.      Meanwhile prepare the white sauce:
5.      Heat a saucepan on a medium heat.
6.      Add the butter to the pan on the side nearest to the handle.
7.      Tilt the pan towards you and allow the butter to melt, whilst trying not to let it cover the rest of the pan.
8.      Now add the flour to the opposite side of the pan and gradually mix the flour into the butter - continue to mix until smooth.

9.      Add the milk and mix thoroughly for 10 minutes until lumps dissolve.
10.     Add pepper.
11.     Turn off the heat and place to one side.
12.     Layer an oven proof lasagna dish with 1/3 eggplant slices.
13.     Add 1/3 beef mince on top.
14.     Layer with 1/3 white sauce.
15.     Repeat until ingredients are used.
16.     Cover and add to the oven for 25-30 minutes or until golden and bubbly.
17.     Remove and serve piping hot!
**Per Serving:** Calories 223
Protein 16 g
Carbohydrates 16 g
Fat 11 g
Sodium 52 mg
Potassium 324 mg
Phosphorus 161 mg

# Chili Beef Strips & Pineapple Salsa
**SERVES 4 / PREP TIME: 5 MINUTES / COOK TIME: 15 MINUTES**

Spice things up in the kitchen.

2 tbsp extra virgin olive oil
1 red onion, diced
1/2 red bell pepper, diced
1 garlic clove, minced
1 red chili, finely diced
6 oz lean beef, cut into strips
f
for the salsa:
1/2 red onion, finely diced
1/2 lime, juiced
1 tbsp fresh cilantro
1/4 cup canned pineapple, diced

2 cups cooked brown rice

1.      Add 1 tbsp oil to a hot pan or skillet over a medium-high heat.

2.      Add 1 onion, pepper, chili and garlic and sauté for 5 minutes until soft.

3.      Add the beef to the pan and stir until browned.

4.      Cook for a further 5-10 minutes or until beef is cooked through.

5.      Prepare the salsa by mixing the rest of the onion, lime juice, cilantro and pineapple.

6.      Serve the beef strips on a bed of rice with the pineapple salsa.

**Per Serving:** Calories 417

Protein 18 g

Carbohydrates 58 g

Fat 10 g

Sodium 27 mg

Potassium 313 mg

Phosphorus 123 mg

# Beef & Ginger Noodles

## SERVES 4 / PREP TIME: 5 MINUTES / COOK TIME: 15 MINUTES

A delicious wok-cooked meal.

1 cup rice noodles

1 tsp coconut oil

6 oz lean frying beef, cut into strips

1 garlic clove, minced

1 tbsp ginger, minced

1 tsp Chinese 5 spice

1/4 cup water chestnuts

1/4 cup green onions, diced

1.      Prepare the noodles according to package guidelines.

2.      Meanwhile, heat the oil in a wok or skillet over a high heat.

3.      Sauté the beef for 5-10 minutes, turning once to brown each side.
4.      Add the garlic and ginger to the pan and sauté for a 2-3 minutes until aromas are released.
5.      Now add the spices and water chestnuts and sauté over a medium heat for 15 minutes or until the beef is soft.
6.      Serve the beef over the noodles and sprinkle with the green onions.
7.      Enjoy!
**Per Serving:** Calories 215
Protein 18 g
Carbohydrates 31 g
Fat 6 g
Sodium 137 mg
Potassium 308 mg
Phosphorus 106 mg

# Apricot & Lamb Stew

**SERVES 2 / PREP TIME: 5 MINUTES / COOK TIME: 1 HOUR & 15 MINUTES**

Supreme!

1 tbsp of olive oil
4oz lean lamb fillets, cubed
1 onion, chopped
2 carrots, diced
1 cup of low sodium chicken broth
1 tsp dried rosemary
3 cups water
1/2 cup canned apricots,juices drained
1 tsp of chopped parsley
1.      In a large casserole dish, heat the olive oil on a medium-high heat.
2.      Add the lamb and cook for 5 minutes until browned.
3.      Add the chopped onion and carrots.

4.     Leave to cook for another 5 minutes until the vegetables begin to soften.

5.     Add the chicken broth and rosemary.

6.     Then cover the casserole and leave to simmer on a low heat for 1 hour until the lamb is tender and fully cooked through.

7.     Add the apricots 20 minutes before serving time.

8.     Plate up and serve with the chopped parsley to garnish.

9.     Hint: You can do this in a pan and then transfer to a slow cooker to leave overnight if you prefer!

**Per Serving:** Calories 118

Protein 8 g

Carbohydrates 13 g

Fat 5 g

Sodium 180 mg

Potassium 254 mg

Phosphorus 157 mg

# Beef And Turnip Stroganoff

**SERVES 2 / PREP TIME: 10 MINUTES / COOK TIME: 4-5 HOURS IN CROCK POT**

A kidney-friendly take on the classic!

1 tbsp black pepper

1 tsp dried oregano

1 garlic clove, minced

1/2 onion, diced

2 turnips, peeled and diced

1 cup low salt chicken or vegetable stock

1 cup water

4 oz stewing beef, diced

1/2 cup almond milk

1/4 cup plain flour

1 cup brown rice

1/4 cup fresh parsley, chopped

1.    In a crock-pot or slow cooker, add the pepper, oregano, garlic, onion, turnips, stock, water and beef.
2.    Cover and cook on high for 4-5 hours or until beef is tender.
3.    Add the flour and almond milk to the crock pot and mix until smooth.
4.    Continue to cook for another 20 minutes or until the mixture has thickened.
5.    Meanwhile, bring a pan of water to the boil and add the rice for 20 minutes.
6.    Drain the water from the rice, add the lid and steam for 5 minutes.
7.    Serve the rice with the creamy beef over the top and garnish with the fresh parsley.

**Per Serving:** Calories 487

Protein 23 g

Carbohydrates 68 g

Fat 13 g

Sodium 126 mg

Potassium 351 mg

Phosphorus 225 mg

# Red Thai Curry

**SERVES 4 / PREP TIME: 10 MINUTES / COOK TIME: 50 MINUTES**

A sensational lamb curry.

1 tbsp fresh basil leaves

1 red chili, diced

1 red bell pepper, diced

1/2 stick lemon grass, chopped

1 tbsp coconut oil

7oz lean lamb, cubed

1/2 white onion, diced

1 garlic clove, minced

1/2 cup almond/rice milk

1/2 cup water

2 cups cooked brown rice

1.      Blend the chili, red pepper, basil, lemon grass and oil in a blender until a paste is formed. Alternatively use a pestle and mortar.

2.      Heat a wok or skillet over a medium to high heat.

3.      Spray a little cooking spray into the pan and add the lamb breasts for 5 minutes on each side or until brown.

4.      Add the onions and garlic and sauté for 3 minutes.

5.      Now pour the rice milk, stock and paste into the pan and stir until it dissolves.

6.      Allow to simmer on a medium to low heat for 30-40 minutes or until lamb is soft.

7.      Serve with the brown rice.

**Per Serving:** Calories 425

Protein 11 g

Carbohydrates 56 g

Fat 15 g

Sodium 68 mg

Potassium 248 mg

Phosphorus 262 mg

# Pork Chops & Rainbow Salad
## SERVES 2 / PREP TIME:5MINUTES / COOK TIME: 10 MINUTES

So simple yet so delicious!

2x 3oz pork chops, fat trimmed

1 tsp black pepper

1 tsp smoked paprika

1/4 cup scallions, sliced

1/4 red bell pepper, diced

1/4 green bell pepper, diced

1/4 cup corn

1 tsp dried tarragon

1 tbsp olive oil

1.      Preheat the broiler or grill to a medium-high heat.
2.      Sprinkle the black pepper and paprika over the pork chops and rub.
3.      Broil or grill the chops for 10-12 minutes or according to package directions.
4.      Meanwhile, mix the vegetables with the oil and tarragon.
5.      Serve the pork chops with the rainbow salad on the side.

**Per Serving:** Calories 298
Protein 22 g
Carbohydrates 8 g
Fat 19 g
Sodium 196 mg
Potassium 410 mg
Phosphorus 225 mg

# Rutabaga & Turnip Cottage Pie
## SERVES 6/ PREP TIME: 10 MINUTES / COOK TIME: 1 HOUR

A kidney friendly version of the British staple.

1 cup rutabaga, peeled & sliced
1 turnip, peeled and sliced
1 tsp olive oil
1 onion, diced
2 carrots, peeled & diced
12 oz lean ground beef
1 tsp black pepper

1.      Preheat the oven to 350°f/170°c/Gas Mark 4.
2.      Bring a pot of water to the boil and add the rutabaga.
3.      Turn down the heat slightly and allow to simmer for 20 minutes.
4.      Add the turnip to this pan in the last 10 minutes.
5.      Meanwhile, add the oil to a pan on a medium heat.
6.      Add the onions and sauté for 4-5 minutes or until soft.
7.      Now add the carrots and sauté for a further 5 minutes.
8.      Add the ground beef and mix until beef is browned.

9.	Add the water, turn the heat to high until it starts to bubble and then reduce the heat and add the thyme and black pepper.

10.	Remove from the heat and check that the rutabaga and turnips are soft with a fork.

11.	Drain and mash with a potato masher.

12.	Pour the beef mixture into a rectangular oven dish.

13.	Top with the mash.

14.	Use your fork to gently score the top of the mash, creating soft lines along the top.

15.	Add to the oven for 30-40 minutes or until golden brown.

16.	Remove and serve immediately!

**Per Serving:** Calories 132

Protein 12 g

Carbohydrates 7 g

Fat 6 g

Sodium 62 mg

Potassium 409 mg

Phosphorus 134 mg

# Egg Fried Rice & Beef

**SERVES 4 / PREP TIME: 5 MINUTES / COOK TIME: 10-15 MINUTES**

Ready in a flash!

1 tbsp coconut oil

8oz lean beef strips

1/4 cup cauliflower florets, thinly sliced

1 cup cooked white rice

2 egg whites

1/4 cup scallions, sliced

pinch black pepper

1.	Heat the oil in a wok or pan over a medium-high heat.

2.	Add the beef strips and cook, turning only once half way through for 8-10 minutes or depending on package guidelines.

3. Add the cauliflower slices to the pan and sauté for 3-4 minutes.
4. Remove the beef and cauliflower and place to one side.
5. Now add the rice to the wok and lower the heat.
6. Quickly, stir in the egg whites until combined with the rice.
7. Serve the beef and cauliflower on a bed of rice.
8. Scatter the scallions over the top.
9. Add black pepper to taste.

**Per Serving:** Calories 207
Protein 25 g
Carbohydrates 12 g
Fat 25 g
Sodium 64 mg
Potassium 254 mg
Phosphorus 162 mg

# Vegetarian & vegan

## Thai Tofu Broth

**SERVES 4 / PREP TIME: 5 MINUTES / COOK TIME: 15 MINUTES**

Tasty tofu with Thai flavors.

1 tbsp coconut oil
6oz drained, pressed and cubed tofu
1/2 onion, sliced
1/2 cup rice milk
1/2 cup water
1 cup rice noodles
1/2 chili, finely sliced
1/2 cup canned water chestnuts
1 cup of snow peas
1 tbsp lime juice
1/4 cup scallions, sliced

1.	Heat the oil in a wok on a high heat and then sauté the tofu until brown on each side.
2.	Add the onion and sauté for 2-3 minutes.
3.	Add the rice milk and water to the wok until bubbling.
4.	Lower to a medium heat and add the noodles, chili and water chestnuts.
5.	Allow to simmer for 10-15 minutes and then add the sugar snap peas for 5 minutes.
6.	Serve with a sprinkle of scallions.
**Per Serving:** Calories 304
Protein 9 g
Carbohydrates 38 g
Fat 13 g
Sodium 36 mg
Potassium 114 mg
Phosphorus 101 mg

## Delicious Vegetarian Lasagne
**SERVES 4 / PREP TIME: 10 MINUTES / COOK TIME: 1 HOUR**

Tastes just as good without the meat!

1/2 zucchini , sliced
1/2 red pepper, sliced
1 cup eggplant, sliced
1 cup of rice milk
1/2 pack of soft tofu
1 tbsp olive oil
1/2 red onion, diced
1 garlic clove, minced
1 tsp oregano
1 tsp basil
a pinch of black pepper to taste
3 lasagna sheets
1.	Preheat oven to 325°F/170 °C/Gas Mark 3.
2.	Slice zucchini, eggplant and pepper into vertical strips.

3.      Add the rice milk and tofu to a food processor and blitz until smooth. Place to one side.

4.      Heat the oil in a skillet over a medium heat and add the onions and garlic for 3-4 minutes or until soft.

5.      Sprinkle in the herbs and pepper and allow to stir through for 5-6 minutes until hot.

6.      Into a lasagne or suitable oven dish, layer 1 lasagna sheet, then 1/3 the eggplant, followed by 1/3 zucchini, then 1/3 pepper before pouring over 1/3 of tofu white sauce.

7.      Repeat for the next 2 layers, finishing with the white sauce.

8.      Add to the oven for 40-50 minutes or until veg is soft and can easily by sliced into servings.

**Per Serving:** Calories 235

Protein 5 g

Carbohydrates 10g

Fat 9 g

Sodium 35 mg

Potassium 129 mg

Phosphorus 66 mg

# Chili Tofu Noodles

## SERVES 4 / PREP TIME: 5 MINUTES / COOK TIME: 15 MINUTES

Packs a punch!

1 cup green beans

2 cups rice noodles

1 tbsp coconut oil

6oz silken firm tofu, pressed & cubed

1/2 red chili, finely diced

1 garlic clove, minced

1 tsp fresh ginger, grated

1/2 lime, juiced

1.      Steam the green beans for 10-12 minutes or according to package directions and drain.

2.    Cook the noodles in a pot of boiling water for 10-15 minutes or according to package directions.

3.    Meanwhile, heat a wok or skillet on a high heat and add coconut oil.

4.    Now add the tofu, chili flakes, garlic and ginger and sauté for 5-10 minutes.

5.    Drain the noodles and add to the wok along with the green beans and lime juice.

6.    Toss to coat.

7.    Serve hot!

**Per Serving:** Calories 246

Protein 10 g

Carbohydrates 28g

Fat 12 g

Sodium 25 mg

Potassium 126 mg

Phosphorus 79 mg

# Curried Cauliflower

## SERVES 4 / PREP TIME: 5 MINUTES / COOK TIME: 20 MINUTES

Cauliflower is often used in Indian cuisine, due to its chunky texture and health benefits.

1 tbsp coconut oil

1 onion, diced

1 garlic clove, minced

1 tsp cumin

1 tsp turmeric

1 tsp garam masala

1/2 chili, diced

2 cups cauliflower, florets

1/2 cup water

1 tbsp fresh cilantro, chopped to garnish

1.    Add the oil to a skillet on a medium heat.

2.    Sauté the onion and garlic for 5 minutes until soft.

3.      Add the cumin, turmeric and garam masala and stir to release the aromas.

4.      Now add the chili to the pan along with the cauliflower.

5.      Stir to coat.

6.      Pour in the water and reduce the heat to a simmer for 15 minutes.

7.      Garnish with cilantro to serve.

**Per Serving:** Calories 108

Protein 2 g

Carbohydrates 11 g

Fat 7 g

Sodium 35 mg

Potassium 328 mg

Phosphorus 39 mg

# Chinese Tempeh Stir Fry

**SERVES 2 / PREP TIME: 5 MINUTES / COOK TIME: 15 MINUTES**

Quick and easy stir-fry dinner!

1 tbsp coconut oil

1 clove garlic, minced

1 tsp fresh ginger, minced

2oz tempeh, sliced

1/2 cup green onions

1/2 cup corn

1 cup brown rice, cooked

1.      Heat the oil in a skillet or wok on a high heat and add the garlic and ginger.

2.      Sauté for 1 minute.

3.      Now add the tempeh and cook for 5-6 minutes before adding the corn for a further 10 minutes.

4.      Now add the green onions and serve over brown rice.

**Per Serving:** Calories 304

Protein 10 g

Carbohydrates 35 g

Fat 4 g
Sodium 91 mg
Potassium 121 mg
Phosphorus 222 mg

# Parsley Root Veg Stew
**SERVES 4 / PREP TIME: 5 MINUTES / COOK TIME: 35-40 MINUTES**

A vegetarian take on this classic dish.

2 tbsp olive oil
1 onion, diced
4 turnips, peeled and diced
2 cloves of garlic
1 tsp ground cumin
1 tsp ground ginger
1/2 tsp ground cinnamon
1 tsp cayenne pepper
2 carrots, peeled and diced
2 cups water
1/4 cup fresh parsley, chopped
2 cups white rice

1.      In a large pot, heat the oil on a medium high heat before sautéing the onion for 4-5 minutes until soft.
2.      Add the turnips and cook for 10 minutes or until golden brown.
3.      Add the garlic, cumin, ginger, cinnamon, and cayenne pepper, cooking for a further 3 minutes.
4.      Add the carrots and stock to the pot and then bring to the boil.
5.      Turn the heat down to a medium heat, cover and simmer for 20 minutes.
6.      Meanwhile add the rice to a pot of water and bring to the boil.
7.      Turn down to simmer for 15 minutes.

8.      Drain and place the lid on for 5 minutes to steam.

9.      Garnish the root vegetable stew with parsley to serve alongside the rice.

**Per Serving:** Calories 210

Protein 4 g

Carbohydrates 32 g

Fat 7 g

Sodium 67 mg

Potassium 181 mg

Phosphorus 105 mg

# Mixed Pepper Paella

**SERVES 2 / PREP TIME: 10 MINUTES / COOK TIME: 35-40 MINUTES**

A delicious protein packed meal!

1 cup brown rice

1 tbsp extra virgin olive oil

1/2 red bell pepper, chopped

1/2 yellow bell pepper, chopped

1/2 zucchini, chopped

1/2 red onion, chopped

1 tsp paprika

1 tsp oregano (dried)

1 tsp parsley (dried)

1 lemon

1 cup homemade chicken broth

1.      Add the rice to a pot of cold water and cook for 15 minutes.

2.      Drain the water, cover the pan and leave to one side.

3.      Heat the oil in a skillet over a medium-high heat.

4.      Add the bell pepper,s onion and zucchini, sautéing for 5 minutes.

5.      To the pan, add the rice, herbs, spices and juice of the lemon along with the chicken broth.

6.      Cover and turn heat right down and allow to simmer for 15-20 minutes.

7.      Serve hot.

**Per Serving:** Calories 210

Protein 4 g

Carbohydrates 33 g

Fat 7 g

Sodium 20 mg

Potassium 33 mg

Phosphorus 156 mg

# Cauliflower Rice & Runny Eggs

## SERVES 4 / PREP TIME: 5 MINUTES / COOK TIME: 30 MINUTES

Yummy

2 cups cauliflower

1 tbsp extra virgin olive oil

1 tbsp curry powder

4 eggs

1 tsp black pepper

1 tbsp fresh chives, chopped

1.      Preheat the oven to 375°f/190°c/Gas Mark 5.

2.      Soak the cauliflower in warm water in advance if possible.

3.      Grate or chop into rice-size pieces.

4.      Bring the cauliflower to the boil in a pot of water and then turn down to simmer for 7 minutes.

5.      Drain completely.

6.      Place on a baking tray and sprinkle over curry powder and black pepper - toss to coat.

7.      Bake in the oven for 20 minutes, stirring occasionally.

8.      Meanwhile, boil a separate pan of water and add the eggs for 7 minutes.

9.      Run under the cold tap, crack and peel the eggs before cutting in half.

10. Top the cauliflower with eggs and chopped chives.
11. Serve hot!

**Per Serving:** Calories 120

Protein 7 g

Carbohydrates 4 g

Fat 8 g

Sodium 175 mg

Potassium 188 mg

Phosphorus 134 mg

# Minted Zucchini Noodles

**SERVES 2 / PREP TIME: 5 MINUTES / COOK TIME: 10 MINUTES**

Fresh and light noodles with an lemony arugula topping.

1/2 cup fresh mint, chopped

1 tsp black pepper

1/4 red chili, de-seeded and chopped

2 tbsp extra virgin olive oil1

4 zucchinis, peeled and sliced

vertically to make noodles (use a spiralizer)

1/2 cup arugula

1/2 lemon, juiced

1. Whisk the mint, pepper, chili and olive oil to make a dressing.
2. Meanwhile, heat a pan of water on a high heat and bring to the boil.
3. Add the zucchini noodles and turn the heat down to simmer for 3-4 minutes.
4. Remove from the heat and place in a bowl of cold water immediately.
5. Toss the noodles in the dressing.
6. Mix the arugula with the lemon juice to serve on the top.
7. Enjoy!

**Per Serving:** Calories 148

Protein 2 g

Carbohydrates 4 g
Fat 13 g
Sodium 7 mg
Potassium 422 mg
Phosphorus 256 mg

# Chili Tempeh & Scallions

**SERVES 2 / PREP TIME: 10 MINUTES / COOK TIME: 15 MINUTES**
Chunky tempeh with a kick.

1 tsp coconut oil
1 tsp soy sauce
1 lime, juiced
1 tbsp ginger, grated
1/2 red chili, de-seeded and chopped
2oz tempeh, cubed
1/2 cup scallions, chopped
1.    Mix the oil, soy sauce, chili flakes, lime juice and ginger together.
2.    Marinate the tempeh in this for as long as possible.
3.    Preheat the broiler to a medium heat.
4.    Add tempeh to a lined baking tray and broil for 10-15 minutes or until hot through.
5.    Remove and sprinkle with scallions to serve.
**Per Serving:** Calories 221
Protein 6 g
Carbohydrates 8 g
Fat 10 g
Sodium 466 mg
Potassium 189 mg
Phosphorus 99 mg

# Seafood

## Shrimp Paella

**SERVES 2 / PREP TIME: 5 MINUTES / COOK TIME: 10 MINUTES**

Tasty seafood dish.

1 tbsp olive oil
1 red onion, chopped
1 garlic clove, chopped
6 oz frozen cooked shrimp
1 tsp paprika
1 chili pepper, de-seeded and sliced
1 tbsp oregano
1 cup cooked brown rice

1.      Heat the olive oil in a large pan on a medium-high heat.
2.      Add the onion and garlic and sauté for 2-3 minutes until soft.
3.      Now add the shrimp and sauté for a further 5 minutes or until hot through.
4.      Now add the herbs,spices, chili and rice with 1/2 cup boiling water.
5.      Stir until everything is warm and the water has been absorbed.
6.      Plate up and serve.

**Per Serving:** Calories 221
Protein 17 g
Carbohydrates 31 g
Fat 8 g
Sodium 235 mg

Potassium 176 mg
Phosphorus 189 mg

# Salmon & Pesto Salad
## SERVES 2 / PREP TIME: 5 MINUTES / COOK TIME: 15 MINUTES

Add a little twist to your normal salmon dish.

For the pesto:
1/2 cup fresh basil
1/2 cup fresh arugula
1 tsp black pepper
1/4 cup extra virgin olive oil
1 garlic clove, minced
For the salmon:
1 tbsp coconut oil
4oz salmon fillet, skinless

For the salad:
1/2 cup iceberg lettuce, washed
2 radishes, sliced
1/2 lemon, juiced
1 tsp black pepper

1.      Prepare the pesto by blending all the ingredients for the pesto in a food processor or by grinding with a pestle and mortar.
2.      Place to one side.
3.      Add a skillet to the stove on a medium-high heat and melt the coconut oil.
4.      Add the salmon to the pan.
5.      Cook for 7-8 minutes and turn over.
6.      Cook for a further 3-4 minutes or until cooked through.
7.      Remove fillets from the skillet and allow to rest.
8.      Mix the lettuce and the radishes and squeeze over juice of 1/2 lemon.
9.      Flake the salmon with a fork and mix through the salad.

10.	Toss to coat and sprinkle with a little black pepper to serve.
**Per Serving:** Calories 221
Protein 13 g
Carbohydrates 1 g
Fat 34 g
Sodium 80 mg
Potassium 119 mg
Phosphorus 158 mg

# Baked Fennel & Garlic Sea Bass
## SERVES 2 / PREP TIME: 5 MINUTES / COOK TIME: 15 MINUTES

Juicy and flavorsome,

1 tsp black pepper
2x 3oz sea bass fillets
1/2 fennel bulb, sliced
2 garlic cloves
1 lemon
1.	Preheat the oven to 375°f/190°c/Gas Mark 5.
2.	Sprinkle black pepper over the Sea Bass.
3.	Slice the fennel bulb and garlic cloves.
4.	Add 1 salmon fillet and half the fennel and garlic to one sheet of baking paper or tin foil.
5.	Squeeze in 1/2 lemon juices.
6.	Repeat for the other fillet.
7.	Fold and add to the oven for 12-15 minutes or until fish is thoroughly cooked through.
8.	Meanwhile, add boiling water to your couscous, cover and allow to steam.
9.	Serve with your choice of rice or salad.
**Per Serving:** Calories 221
Protein 14 g
Carbohydrates 3 g
Fat 2 g

Sodium 119 mg
Potassium 398 mg
Phosphorus 149 mg

# Lemon, Garlic & Cilantro Tuna And Rice
**SERVES 2 / PREP TIME: 5 MINUTES / COOK TIME: NA**

Prepare in advance for a go-to lunch!

3oz canned tuna in water
1 tbsp extra virgin olive oil
1 tsp black pepper
2 tbsp fresh cilantro, chopped
1/4 red onion, finely diced
1 lemon, juiced
1 cup rice, cooked
1/2 cup arugula, washed

1.      Mix the olive oil, pepper, cilantro and red onion in a bowl.
2.      Stir in the tuna , cover and leave in the fridge for as long as possible (if you can) or serve immediately.
3.      When ready to eat, serve up with the cooked rice and arugula!

**Per Serving:** Calories 221
Protein 11 g
Carbohydrates 26 g
Fat 7 g
Sodium 143 mg
Potassium 197 mg
Phosphorus 182 mg

# Cod & Green Bean Risotto
**SERVES 2 / PREP TIME: 4 MINUTES / COOK TIME: 40 MINUTES**

Soft and succulent lemon-infused fish risotto.

1 tbsp extra virgin olive oil

1 white onion, finely diced

1 cup white rice

1 cup low sodium chicken broth (see soups and stocks chapter)

1 cup boiling water

1/2 cup of green beans

4oz cod fillet

pinch of black pepper

2 lemon wedges

1/2 cup arugula

1. Heat the oil in a large pan on a medium heat.

2. Sauté the chopped onion for 5 minutes until soft before adding in the rice and stirring for 1-2 minutes.

3. Combine the broth with boiling water.

4. Add half of the liquid to the pan and stir slowly.

5. Slowly add the rest of the liquid whilst continuously stirring for up to 20-30 minutes.

6. Stir in the green beans to the risotto.

7. Place the fish on top of the rice, cover and steam for 10 minutes.

8. Ensure the water does not dry out and keep topping up until the rice is cooked thoroughly.

9. Use your fork to break up the fish fillets and stir into the rice.

10. Sprinkle with freshly ground pepper to serve and a squeeze of fresh lemon.

11. Garnish with the lemon wedges and serve with the arugula.

**Per Serving:** Calories 221

Protein 12 g

Carbohydrates 29 g

Fat 8 g

Sodium 398 mg

Potassium 347 mg

Phosphorus 241 mg

# Mixed Pepper Stuffed River Trout
## SERVES 4 / PREP TIME: 5 MINUTES / COOK TIME: 20 MINUTES

This tastes scrumptious and fresh!

1 tsp extra virgin olive oil
1/4 red pepper, diced
1/4 yellow pepper, diced
1/4 green pepper, diced
1 tsp thyme
1 tsp oregano
1 tsp black pepper
1 lime, juiced
1 whole river trout (8oz), skinned and gutted by your fishmonger
1 cup baby spinach leaves, washed

1. Preheat the broiler /grill on a high heat.
2. Lightly oil a baking tray.
3. Mix all of the ingredients apart from the trout and lime.
4. Slice the trout lengthways (there should be an opening here from where it was gutted) and stuff the mixed ingredients inside.
5. Squeeze the lime juice over the fish and then place the lime wedges on the tray.
6. Place under the broiler on the baking tray and broil for 15-20 minutes or until fish is thoroughly cooked through and flakes easily.
7. Enjoy alone or with a side helping of rice or salad.

**Per Serving:** Calories 290
Protein 15 g
Carbohydrates 0 g
Fat 7 g
Sodium 43 mg
Potassium 315 mg
Phosphorus 189 mg

# Haddock & Buttered Leeks

**SERVES 2 / PREP TIME: 5 MINUTES / COOK TIME: 15 MINUTES**

A simple yet divine recipe

2x 3oz haddock fillets
A pinch of black pepper
1/2 lemon, juiced
1 tbsp unsalted butter
1 leek, sliced widthways
2 tsp parsley, chopped

1.      Preheat the oven to 375°f/190°c/Gas Mark 5.
2.      Add the haddock fillets to baking or parchment paper and sprinkle with the black pepper.
3.      Squeeze over the lemon juice and wrap into a parcel.
4.      Bake the parcel on a baking tray for 10-15 minutes or until fish is thoroughly cooked through.
5.      Meanwhile, heat the butter over a medium-low heat in a small pan.
6.      Add the leeks and parsley and sauté for 5-7 minutes until soft.
7.      Serve the haddock fillets on a bed of buttered leeks and enjoy!

**Per Serving:** Calories 124
Protein 15 g
Carbohydrates 0 g
Fat 7 g
Sodium 161 mg
Potassium 251 mg
Phosphorus 220 mg

# Thai Spiced Halibut

**SERVES 2 PREP TIME: 5 MINUTES COOK TIME: 20 MINUTES**

Bring a taste of Thailand to your dinner table.

4oz halibut fillet

A pinch of black pepper

2 garlic cloves, pressed

2 tbsp coconut oil

1 lime, halved

1/2 red chilli, diced

2 green onions, sliced

1 lime leaf

1 tbsp fresh basil

1 cup of white rice

1.      Preheat oven to 400°f/190°c/Gas Mark 5.

2.      Add half of the ingredients into baking paper and fold into a parcel.

3.      Repeat for your second parcel.

4.      Add to the oven for 15-20 minutes or until fish is thoroughly cooked through.

5.      Serve with cooked rice.

**Per Serving:** Calories 311

Protein 16 g

Carbohydrates 17 g

Fat 15 g

Sodium 31 mg

Potassium 418 mg

Phosphorus 257 mg

# CONVERSION TABLES

**Volume**

| Imperial | Metric |
|---|---|
| 1 tbsp | 15ml |
| 2 fl oz | 55 ml |
| 3 fl oz | 75 ml |
| 5 fl oz (¼ pint) | 150 ml |
| 10 fl oz (½ pint) | 275 ml |
| 1 pint | 570 ml |
| 1 ¼ pints | 725 ml |

| | |
|---|---|
| 1 ¾ pints | 1 litre |
| 2 pints | 1.2 litres |
| 2½ pints | 1.5 litres |
| 4 pints | 2.25 litres |

**Weight**

| Imperial | Metric |
|---|---|
| ½ oz | 10 g |
| ¾ oz | 20 g |
| 1 oz | 25 g |
| 1½ oz | 40 g |
| 2 oz | 50 g |
| 2½ oz | 60 g |
| 3 oz | 75 g |
| 4 oz | 110 g |
| 4½ oz | 125 g |
| 5 oz | 150 g |
| 6 oz | 175 g |
| 7 oz | 200 g |
| 8 oz | 225 g |
| 9 oz | 250 g |
| 10 oz | 275 g |
| 12 oz | 350 g |
| 1 lb | 450 g |
| 1 lb 8 oz | 700 g |

| 2 lb | 900 g |
|------|-------|
| 3 lb | 1.35 kg |

## Metric cups conversion

| Cups | Imperial | Metric |
|------|----------|--------|
| 1 cup flour | 5oz | 150g |
| 1 cup caster or granulated sugar | 8oz | 225g |
| 1 cup soft brown sugar | 6oz | 175g |
| 1 cup soft butter/margarine | 8oz | 225g |
| 1 cup sultanas/raisins | 7oz | 200g |
| 1 cup currants | 5oz | 150g |
| 1 cup ground almonds | 4oz | 110g |
| 1 cup oats | 4oz | 110g |
| 1 cup golden syrup/honey | 12oz | 350g |
| 1 cup uncooked rice | 7oz | 200g |
| 1 cup grated cheese | 4oz | 110g |
| 1 stick butter | 4oz | 110g |
| ¼ cup liquid (water, milk, oil etc) | 4 tablespoons | 60ml |
| ½ cup liquid (water, milk, oil etc) | ¼ pint | 125ml |
| 1 cup liquid (water, milk, oil etc) | ½ pint | 250ml |
| | | |

## Oven temperatures

| Gas Mark | Fahrenheit | Celsius |
|----------|------------|---------|
| 1/4 | 225 | 110 |
| 1/2 | 250 | 130 |

| 1 | 275 | 140 |
|---|-----|-----|
| 2 | 300 | 150 |
| 3 | 325 | 170 |
| 4 | 350 | 180 |
| 5 | 375 | 190 |
| 6 | 400 | 200 |
| 7 | 425 | 220 |
| 8 | 450 | 230 |
| 9 | 475 | 240 |

**Oven temperatures**

| Gas Mark | Fahrenheit | Celsius |
|----------|------------|---------|
| 1/4 | 225 | 110 |
| 1/2 | 250 | 130 |
| 1 | 275 | 140 |
| 2 | 300 | 150 |
| 3 | 325 | 170 |
| 4 | 350 | 180 |
| 5 | 375 | 190 |
| 6 | 400 | 200 |
| 7 | 425 | 220 |
| 8 | 450 | 230 |
| 9 | 475 | 240 |

**Weight**

| Imperial | Metric |
|----------|--------|
| ½ oz | 10 g |
| ¾ oz | 20 g |
| 1 oz | 25 g |

| | |
|---|---|
| 1½ oz | 40 g |
| 2 oz | 50 g |
| 2½ oz | 60 g |
| 3 oz | 75 g |
| 4 oz | 110 g |
| 4½ oz | 125 g |
| 5 oz | 150 g |
| 6 oz | 175 g |
| 7 oz | 200 g |
| 8 oz | 225 g |
| 9 oz | 250 g |
| 10 oz | 275 g |
| 12 oz | 350 g |
| 1 lb | 450 g |
| 1 lb 8 oz | 700 g |
| 2 lb<br>3 lb | 900 g<br>1.35 kg |

# Part 2

# Chapter 1

# The renal diet

A renal diet is just a diet that has been recommended for somebody with kidney illness that depends on the phase of kidney sickness, blood work results, drugs and some other dietary needs. Since there is no standard renal diet, the diet can shift from individual to individual and can change after some time. The objectives of the diet are intricate. However, it can be separated, all things considered:

- _To stop the development of the poisons that healthy kidneys ordinarily get out of the blood._

- _To lessen the remaining task at hand of the kidneys before dialysis._

- _To counteract intricacies that can happen from a development of poisons._

- _To meet all your wholesome needs._

While the diet might be distinctive for everybody, the normal components are confined sodium, potassium, phosphorus, and low or high protein. A few people may require a liquid limitation too. An enlisted dietitian will devise a nourishment care plan that is individualized to meet your specific needs.

## How does what I eat and drink influence my hemodialysis?

97

Your decisions about what to eat and drink while on hemodialysis can have any kind of effect by the way you feel and can make your medications work better.

Between dialysis treatment sessions, wastes can develop in your blood and make you weak. You can lessen waste development by controlling what you eat and drink. You can coordinate what you eat and drink with what your kidney medicines remove.

A few nourishments cause wastes to develop immediately between your dialysis sessions. In the event that your blood contains an excessive amount of waste, your kidney treatment session may not remove them all.

How might I realize what I ought to eat?

Your dialysis focus has a renal dietitian to enable you to plan your dinners. A renal dietitian has exceptional skills in thinking about the nourishment and sustenance needs of individuals with kidney sickness.

Utilize this data to enable you to figure out how to eat right when on hemodialysis. Peruse each area in turn. At that point, review with your renal dietitian, the segments checked.

Keep a duplicate of this data to help yourself remember nourishments you can eat and food sources to avoid.

Dietitian speaking with couple. Meet with a renal dietitian to make an eating plan that will function admirably for you.

Do I have to watch what I eat and drink?

Definitely. You should cautiously plan your suppers and monitor the amount of fluids you consume. It is best to stay away from nourishments and refreshments that have loads of:

- *potassium*

- *phosphorus*

- *sodium—for instance, vegetable squeeze and sports drinks*

For what reason is it essential to monitor what amount of fluid I eat or drink?

You may feel good on the off chance that you monitor how much fluid you eat and drink. Overabundance of liquid can develop in your body and may cause:

- *growing and weight gain between dialysis sessions*

- *changes in your pulse*

- *your heart has to work more harder, which can prompt genuine heart issues*

- *a development of liquid in your lungs, making it difficult for you to relax*

Hemodialysis expels additional liquid from your body. Notwithstanding, hemodialysis can remove just such a great amount of liquid at a time securely. On the off chance that you go to your hemodialysis with an excess of liquid in your body, your treatment may make you feel sick. You may get muscle spasms or have an abrupt drop in pulse that makes you feel woozy or wiped out to your stomach.

Your social insurance supplier can enable you to make sense of how a lot of fluid is directly for you.

One approach to restrict how a lot of fluid you have is to reduce the salt in the nourishments you eat. Salt makes you parched, so you drink more. It is best to avoid salty nourishments, for example, chips and pretzels.

Your renal dietitian will give you different tips to enable you to control how a lot of fluid you expend while ensuring you don't feel excessively parched.

What nourishments consider fluid and why?

Nourishments that are fluid at room temperature, for example, soup, contain water. Gelatin, pudding, frozen yogurt, and different nourishments that incorporate a great deal of fluid in the formula are like this as well. Most foods grown from the ground contain water, for example, melons, grapes, apples, oranges, tomatoes, lettuce, and celery. When you check up how much fluid you have in a day, make certain to tally these nourishments.

Bowl of chicken soup. Any nourishment that is fluid at room temperature contains water. A few nourishments, as most foods grown from the ground, are not fluid at room temperature but also add to the absolute fluid quantity you eat.

What is my dry weight?

Your dry weight is your weight after a hemodialysis session has expelled all additional liquid from your body. Controlling your fluid admission encourages you to remain at your appropriate dry weight. In the event that you let an excessive amount of liquid develop between sessions, it is much harder to accomplish your dry weight. Your health provider can enable you to make sense of what dry weight is directly for you.

What do I have to think about potassium?

Solid kidneys keep the perfect amount of potassium in your blood to keep your heart thumping at an unfaltering pace. Potassium levels can ascend between hemodialysis sessions and influence your pulse. Eating a lot of potassium can be risky to your heart and may even cause death.

To control potassium levels, limit potassium-rich nourishments, for example, avocados, bananas, kiwis, and dried organic product. Pick products of the soil that are lower in potassium. Have little parts of nourishments that are higher in potassium, for example, a couple of cherry tomatoes on a plate of mixed greens or a couple of raisins in your cereal.

You can expel a portion of the potassium from potatoes by dicing or destroying them and after that bubbling them in a full pot of water.

To expel a portion of the potassium from potatoes:

Shakers potatoes into little pieces.

Individual grinding potatoes or grind potatoes into shreds.

Diced potatoes bubbling in a pot of water and then bubble potatoes in a full pot of water.

Your renal dietitian will give you increasingly explicit data about the potassium substance of nourishments.

# Converse with Your Renal Dietitian

Make a nourishment arrangement that lessens the potassium in your diet. Start by taking note of the high-potassium nourishments you presently eat. Your renal dietitian can enable you to add nourishments to the rundown.

Changes

about nourishments you can eat rather than high-potassium nourishments.

Rather than _____, I can eat _____.

Rather than _____, I can eat _____.

Rather than _____, I can eat _____.

Rather than _____, I can eat _____.

More data is given in the NIDDK wellbeing point, Potassium: Tips for People with Chronic Kidney Disease.

# What do I have to think about phosphorus?

An excessive amount of phosphorus in your blood pulls calcium from your bones. Losing calcium may make your bones powerless and prone to break. Additionally, a lot of phosphorus may make your skin tingle. Controlling phosphorus can be hard on the grounds that nourishments that contain phosphorus, for example, meat and milk, likewise contain the protein you need. You ought to be mindful so as to eat enough protein in any case, less that you get an excessive amount of phosphorus. Handled and bundled nourishments contain particularly elevated levels of phosphorus. You can likewise discover phosphorus normally in nourishments, for example, poultry, fish, nuts, nutty spread, beans, cola, tea, and dairy items. For the most part, individuals on hemodialysis should just have a 1/2 cup of milk for each day. Your renal dietitian will give you progressively explicit data about phosphorus.

You may need to take a phosphate fastener, for example, sevelamer (Renvela), calcium acetic acid derivation (PhosLo), lanthanum carbonate (Fosrenol), or calcium carbonate to control the phosphorus in your blood between hemodialysis sessions. These medications act like plastic packs with zip tops. The phosphorus cover "seals" the phosphorus from nourishment and moves it out through stool so the phosphorous doesn't enter the circulatory system.

Restricting phosphorus and getting enough protein can be troublesome. See the "Chat with Your Renal Dietitian" area under the following segment about protein.

More data is given in the NIDDK wellbeing subject, Phosphorus: Tips for People with Chronic Kidney Disease.

## What do I have to think about protein?

Renal dietitians energize the vast majority on hemodialysis to eat top notch protein since it delivers less waste for expulsion during dialysis. Great protein originates from meat, poultry, fish, and eggs. Keep away from prepared meats, for example, wieners and canned bean stew, which have high amounts of sodium and phosphorus.

Fish, hamburger, chicken, eggs. Renal dietitians support a great many people on hemodialysis to eat top notch protein.

103

About the meats you eat.

I will eat _____ serving(s) of meat every day. A normal serving size is 3 ounces, about the size of the palm of your hand or a deck of cards.

Attempt to pick lean, or low-fat, meats that are low in phosphorus, for example, chicken, fish, or meal hamburger. In the event that you are a vegan, get some information about different approaches to get protein.

Low-fat milk is a decent wellspring of protein. In any case, milk is high in phosphorus and potassium. Milk additionally adds to your fluid admission. to check whether milk fits into your nourishment plan.

On the off chance that milk is in my nourishment plan, I will drink _____ cup(s) of milk a day.

More data is given in the NIDDK wellbeing subject, Protein: Tips for People with Chronic Kidney Disease.

## What do I have to think about sodium?

Sodium is a piece of salt. Sodium is found in many canned, bundled, solidified and quick nourishments. Sodium is additionally found in numerous sauces, seasonings, and meats. A lot of sodium makes you parched, which makes you drink a lot of fluid.

Attempt to eat new, normally low-sodium nourishments. Search for items marked "low sodium," particularly in canned and solidified nourishments.

Try not to utilize salt substitutes since they contain potassium. about flavors you can use to season your nourishment. Your renal dietitian can enable you to discover flavor mixes without sodium or potassium.

Dried herbs and flavor containers; Flavors you can use to enhance your nourishment.

Your renal dietitian can enable you to discover flavors and low-sodium nourishments you may like. Show them here:

Zest: _____

Zest: _____

Zest: _____

Nourishment: _____

Nourishment: _____

More data is given in the NIDDK wellbeing point, Sodium: Tips for People with Chronic Kidney Disease.

What do I have to think about calories?

All nourishments contain calories, and you need calories for vitality. Numerous individuals on hemodialysis don't have a decent hunger and don't get enough calories. On the off chance that you discover you don't want to eat, speak with your renal dietitian to discover solid approaches to add calories to your diet. Vegetable oils, for example, olive oil, canola oil, and safflower oil—are great sources of calories and are the most advantageous approach to add fat to your diet on the off chance that you have to put on weight. Use them liberally on breads, rice, and noodles if your renal dietitian guides you to add calories to your diet.

Spread and margarines are wealthy in calories; be that as it may, they are mostly immersed fat. Soaked fats and trans fats can obstruct your supply routes. Utilize them less regularly. Delicate margarine that arrives in a tub is superior to stick margarine. Pick a delicate margarine with less immersed and trans fats.

Speak with your renal dietitian about the sorts and amounts of fat you need in your diet. Everybody will have various needs that a renal dietitian can help address.

Hard sweet, sugar, nectar, jam and jam give calories and vitality without fat or including different things that your body needn't bother with. In the case where you have diabetes, be cautious about eating desserts and before adding desserts to your nourishment plan.

Olives and compartment of oil. Vegetable oils, for example, olive oil, canola oil, and safflower oil—are great sources of calories.

In the event that you are overweight, your renal dietitian can work with you to lessen the absolute calories you eat every day.

Everybody's calorie needs are extraordinary. You may need to eliminate calories on the off chance that you are overweight, or you may need to discover approaches to add calories to your diet in the event that you are getting more fit easily.
I will get _____ calories consistently.

More data is given in the NIDDK wellbeing point, Food Label Reading: Tips for People with Chronic Kidney Disease.

Would it be advisable for me to take nutrient and mineral enhancements?

You may not get enough nutrients and minerals in your diet since you need to maintain a strategic distance from such a large number of nourishments. Hemodialysis likewise expels a few nutrients from your body. Your health provider may recommend a nutrient and mineral enhancement planned explicitly for individuals with kidney failure.

Cautioning: Do not take nourishing enhancements you can purchase over the counter. These enhancements may contain nutrients or minerals that are destructive to you. For security reasons, chat with your social insurance supplier before utilizing probiotics, dietary enhancements, or some other drug together with or instead of the treatment your medicinal services supplier endorses.

Lady chatting with drug specialist. Chat with your health provider before utilizing probiotics, dietary enhancements, or some other medication together with or instead of the treatment your social insurance supplier endorses.
More data is given in the NIDDK wellbeing point, Eating Right for Kidney Health: Tips for People with Chronic Kidney Disease.

## The renal eating regimen is prohibitive and difficult to pursue

Why are patients with ceaseless kidney ailment and kidney illness devouring a Western-type diet? On the off chance that you are an enlisted dietitian, you realize that the renal eating routine is one of the hardest to recommend. Furthermore, in many cases a patient with kidney sickness has different comorbidities, for example, diabetes and hypertension, which adds a layer of trouble to the therapeutic sustenance treatment. A few dietitians give a rundown of nourishments that are high in potassium, phosphorus, and sodium. If you investigate the arrangements of nourishments, you rapidly understand that your alternatives are diminished. Likewise, a portion of the cooking strategies to diminish these supplements may require additional time and assets, which could be a hindrance for patients and a weight for their parental figures. This may lead patients to dismiss the proposals and might be reflected in the supplement admission and dietary examples announced.

Also, gain admittance to vivid learning encounters, coordinated effort, and systems administration with the best personalities in sustenance.

The conventional way to deal with the renal eating regimen is developing.

The customary way to deal with the renal eating regimen is starting to change. As of late, the European Renal Association-European Dialysis and Transplantation Association prescribed the Mediterranean eating routine as the dietary example of decision for constant kidney infection patients. Also, "changed" dietary suggestions dependent on simple to-pursue rules have been proposed for hemodialysis patients. In any case, there might be some health providers and nourishment experts who may differ with these proposals. One explanation is that potassium admission might be expanded and a danger of high convergences of potassium in blood, or hyperkalemia, may exceed the advantages of the eating routine generally speaking. Be that as it may, the relationship of dietary potassium and serum potassium in end-arrange kidney sickness patients experiencing hemodialysis treatment is feeble. In addition, with these dietary examples the majority of the phosphorus originates from plant-based nourishments, as the utilization of animal based items is restricted, which gives an advantage as the bioavailability of phosphorus is lower than the animal sources and the utilization of ultra-prepared nourishments is likewise constrained.

The Mediterranean and DASH-style diet have been related with diminished cardiovascular and all-cause mortality in the overall public. In kidney illness, a dietary example that looks like these weight control plans has been related with a 27% decrease in mortality chance. Nonetheless, late outcomes from the DIET-HD worldwide companion of more than 8,000 hemodialysis patients demonstrated that a high adherence to the Mediterranean or DASH-type diet was not related with decreased cardiovascular mortality or all-cause mortality. This examination, in any case, was an observational forthcoming worldwide associate from European nations utilizing a nourishment recurrence poll that uses the British Food Composition Table and, along these lines, there is a restricted generalizability of the outcomes.

## The sustenance rules for patients with incessant kidney malady are being refreshed

An update for the significant sustenance rules for kidney sickness patients (the Kidney Disease Outcomes Quality Initiative [K/DOQI] rules by the National Kidney Foundation) is normal in the not so distant future. Despite the fact that a general focal point of supplement proposals is as yet expected, it isn't known whether a specific dietary example will be suggested following the proposals of the European Renal Association-European Dialysis Transplantation Association. In spite of this, no ifs, ands or buts there is a requirement for imminent, randomized-clinical preliminaries to give evidence of the advantage on results and personal satisfaction with concentrating on dietary examples as opposed to minor supplement confinements.

Dialysis does a portion of the work that your kidneys did when they were solid. In any case, dialysis doesn't fill in just as solid kidneys, and it can't do everything that healthy kidneys do. Some waste and liquid may even now develop in your body, particularly between dialysis medicines. After some time, the additional waste and liquid in your blood can cause heart, bone and other medical issues. In the event that you have kidney failure/ESRD, you should screen the amounts of liquid and certain supplements you take in every day. This can help shield waste and liquid from structure up in your blood and causing issues.

# Chapter 2

# Renal diet and eating routine

Precisely how severe your eating routine ought to be relies upon your treatment plan and other wellbeing concerns. A great many people on dialysis need to constrain:

- *Potassium*

- *Phosphorus*

- *Liquids*

- *Sodium*

- *Potassium*

- *Phosphorus*

- *Liquids*

- *Sodium*

- *Hemodialysis diet*

- *Peritoneal dialysis diet*

- *Exceptional strides for individuals with diabetes*

- *Discover kidney-accommodating plans on Kidney Kitchen*

- *Potassium*

Potassium is a mineral found in practically all nourishments. Your body needs some potassium to make your muscles work, however an excessive amount of potassium can be perilous. Having a lot of potassium in your blood is called hyperkalemia. When you are on dialysis, your potassium level might be excessively low or excessively high. Having close to nothing or an excessive amount of potassium can cause muscle issues, shortcoming and sporadic heartbeat. Having an excess of potassium can cause a coronary failure. Ask your dietitian how much potassium you ought to have every day. Print and utilize this potassium log to monitor how a lot of potassium you take in!

Phosphorus

Phosphorus is a mineral found in numerous nourishments. It works with calcium and nutrient D to keep your bones solid. Healthy kidneys help keep the correct parity of phosphorus in your body. When you are on dialysis, phosphorus can develop in your blood. Having an excessive amount of phosphorus is called hyperphosphatemia. This can prompt bone ailment, which causes powerless bones that break effectively. Restricting the amount of phosphorus you take in can help anticipate this issue. Converse with your dietitian about how much phosphorus you ought to have every day.

Liquids

When you are on dialysis, liquid (water) may develop in your body between medications. A lot of liquid in your body can cause hypertension, growing, inconvenience breathing and cardiovascular breakdown. Having additional liquid in your blood can likewise make your dialysis medicines progressively troublesome. In the event that you have to restrict liquids, you should decrease the amount you drink. You may likewise need to curtail a few nourishments that contain a great deal of water. Soups and nourishments that soften, for example, ice, frozen yogurt and gelatin, have a great deal of water in them. Numerous leafy foods are likewise high in water content. Speak with your dietitian about how much liquid you ought to have every day.

In the event that you are restricting liquid and feel parched, attempt these stunts to extinguish your thirst:

Chew gum

Wash your mouth without gulping. You can keep mouthwash in the cooler and use it as a virus flush for your mouth.

Suck on a bit of ice, mints or hard sweet (make sure to consider the ice liquid, and pick without sugar treats in the event that you have diabetes).

Suck on a shot of reusable ice 3D shape. It feels cold, however doesn't add any liquid to your body.

Sodium

Everybody's body needs some sodium to work effectively. Sodium encourages you keep the perfect amount of liquid in your blood. Healthy kidneys help keep the perfect amount of sodium in your body. At the point when your kidneys are not working, sodium can develop in your blood. At the point when this occurs, your body retains an excess of water. This can make your circulatory strain excessively high and can cause issues during your dialysis medications. Restricting how much sodium you take in every day can help monitor your circulatory strain and help keep your body from clutching an excessive amount of liquid. Converse with your dietitian about how much sodium you ought to have every day, and utilize these tips to reduce sodium in your eating regimen:

Try not to add salt to your nourishment when cooking or at the table. Take a stab at cooking with crisp herbs, lemon squeeze or without salt flavors.

Pick new or solidified vegetables rather than canned vegetables. On the off chance that you do utilize canned vegetables, wash them to remove additional salt before cooking or eating them.

Keep away from handled meats, for example, ham, bacon, frankfurter and lunch meats.

Crunch on new foods grown from the ground instead of wafers or other salty bites.

Maintain a strategic distance from cured nourishments, for example, olives and pickles.

Farthest point high-sodium toppings, for example, soy sauce, BBQ sauce and ketchup.

## Hemodialysis diet

In the event that you are on hemodialysis and have medicines three times each week, you will probably need to avoid potassium, sodium, phosphorus and liquids. This is on the grounds that when your blood is being cleaned just three times each week, there is additional time between medicines for waste and liquid to develop in your blood. You may likewise need to restrict the amount of protein you take in. On the off chance that you do hemodialysis at home, and do your medicines each day, you might have the option to be less exacting with your eating regimen. Converse with your dietitian about making an eating regimen arrangement that is specifically for you.

Peritoneal dialysis diet

In the event that you do peritoneal dialysis (PD), you might have the option to take in somewhat more phosphorus, potassium, sodium and liquid than if you did hemodialysis. You will likewise need to eat more protein. This is on the grounds that PD works throughout day and night to remove waste and liquid from your blood. This prevents the waste and liquid from building up in your blood as it does between hemodialysis medicines. In the event that you do PD, converse with your dietitian about making an eating regimen arrangement that is directly for you.

Extraordinary strides for individuals with diabetes

On the off chance that you have diabetes, work with your dietitian to make an eating routine arrangement that enables you to stay away from the supplements you have to avoid, while likewise controlling your glucose. On the off chance that you do PD, remember that PD arrangement has dextrose in it. Dextrose is a kind of sugar. When you do PD, a portion of the dextrose is taken in by your body. On the off chance that you have diabetes, it is essential to include the dextrose in your PD arrangement as additional sugar in your eating routine. Speak with your health provider or dietitian in the event that you have inquiries regarding dealing with your glucose on the off chance that you do PD.

Discover kidney-accommodating plans on Kidney Kitchen

In Kidney Kitchen, you can bring a profound plunge into what every supplement implies for individuals with kidney sickness, and the amount of basic nourishments these supplements contain. Learn what smart dieting implies for individuals in each phase of kidney illness, including those on dialysis or living with a kidney transplant. Discover plans on Kidney Kitchen.

The appropriate response relies upon what kind of veggie lover you are. It additionally relies upon your degree of kidney capacity and how prohibitive you should be with protein, phosphorus and potassium.

An appropriate renal eating routine is a basic piece of any treatment plan for ceaseless kidney sickness. Albeit a renal eating routine cutoff points protein, regardless you have to eat some great protein consistently.

Being a veggie lover doesn't mean passing up quality protein. There are a lot of good plant sources of proteins. Nonetheless, a veggie lover renal eating routine requires a customized dinner plan from an enlisted dietitian since vegan source of protein additionally contain shifting amounts of potassium and phosphorus. Your dietitian can enable you to pick the correct nourishments in the perfect sums.

Your kidneys are responsible for keeping an excessive amount of potassium and phosphorus from structure up in your blood. So it's critical to have the perfect amount of potassium and phosphorus in your eating routine to abstain from overpowering your kidneys' capacity to keep up healthy levels.

Here's some fundamental data:

116

**Protein.** In the diagram underneath, you'll discover a few instances of great protein hotspots for veggie lovers, however pursue your dietitian's proposals.

**Phosphorus.** On the off chance that phosphorus is a worry, it's ideal to stay away from nourishments high in inorganic phosphate, for example, profoundly prepared food sources. Dairy nourishments are a fundamental wellspring of phosphorus in a run of the mill diet. Dairy items can be supplanted with unenriched rice or soy options. Numerous nondairy plant-based milks and yogurt are currently accessible, however most are enhanced with phosphorus-containing added substances. Peruse fixing records cautiously.

**Potassium.** On the off chance that you have to watch potassium, remember that most of potassium originates from dairy items, leafy foods. By constraining dairy and picking leafy foods that are lower in potassium, you can control your potassium level. Nuts, seeds, lentils and beans additionally can raise potassium whenever eaten normally. Splashing and cooking canned and dried vegetables can extraordinarily diminish the amount of potassium they contain. Some low-sodium nourishments contain potassium chloride, so read names cautiously.

**Sodium.** In the event that you have to reduce sodium intake, cut back on the salt you include during cooking and at the table. Additionally, make certain to check nourishment marks. Many prepared to-eat nourishments, canned beans, vegetarian meats, and soy-and rice-based cheeses are high in sodium.

Your dinner plan ought to likewise incorporate rules for other nutrition types, for example, grains, fats and desserts. A feast plan from an enrolled dietitian will enable you to address your issues for calories and other significant supplements.

# Renal eating regimen

Likewise called: kidney diet, dialysis diet

Wastes in the blood originate from nourishment and fluids that are expended. Individuals with kidney ailment must cling to a renal eating routine to eliminate the amount of waste in their blood. Following a renal eating regimen may likewise support kidney capacity and defer absolute kidney failure.

A renal eating regimen is one that is low in sodium, phosphorous and protein. A renal eating routine highlights the significance of expending excellent protein and controlling liquids. Some renal weight control plans may likewise call for restricted potassium and calcium. Each individual is extraordinary, and hence, a dietitian will work with every patient to think of a renal eating regimen that is customized to their needs.

Your kidneys are bean-molded organs that perform numerous significant capacities.

They're accountable for sifting blood, expelling waste through pee, delivering hormones, adjusting minerals and keeping up liquid parity.

There are many hazard factors for kidney illness. The most well-known are uncontrolled diabetes and hypertension.

Liquor addiction, coronary illness, hepatitis C infection and HIV disease are likewise causes

At the point when the kidneys become harmed and can't work appropriately, liquid can develop in the body and waste can collect in the blood.

In any case, keeping away from or restricting certain nourishments in your eating routine may help decline the aggregation of waste items in the blood, improve kidney capacity and counteract further harm (2Trusted Source).

## The Connection Between Diet and Kidney Disease

Dietary confinements differ based on the phase of kidney issue.

For example, individuals who are in the beginning periods of constant kidney illness will have unexpected dietary confinements in comparison to those with end-arrange renal ailment, or kidney failure.

Those with end-arrange renal illness who require dialysis will likewise have shifting dietary limitations. Dialysis is a kind of treatment that removes additional water and channels waste.

Most of those in the late stages or with end-organize kidney ailment should pursue a kidney-accommodating eating routine to maintain a strategic distance from develop of specific synthetic compounds or supplements in the blood.

In those with constant kidney infection, the kidneys can't sufficiently remove high levels of sodium, potassium and phosphorus. Therefore, they are at higher danger of raised blood levels of these minerals.
A kidney-accommodating eating routine, or a "renal eating regimen," as a rule incorporates restricting sodium and potassium to 2,000 mg for each day and constraining phosphorus to 1,000 mg for every day.

Harmed kidneys may likewise experience difficulty separating the waste results of protein digestion. In this way, people with ceaseless kidney sickness in stages 1–4 may need to confine the amount of protein in their weight control plans (3Trusted Source).

In any case, those with end-organize renal ailment experiencing dialysis have an expanded protein necessity (4Trusted Source).

Here are 17 nourishments that you should almost certainly maintain a strategic distance from on a renal eating routine.

1. Dull Colored Colas

Notwithstanding the calories and sugar that colas give, they likewise contain added substances that contain phosphorus, particularly dull shaded colas.

Numerous nourishment producers include phosphorus during the preparing of nourishment and drinks to improve season, drag out timeframe of realistic usability and counteract staining.

This additional phosphorus is significantly more absorbable by the human body than regular, animal or plant-based phosphorus (5Trusted Source).

In contrast to characteristic phosphorus, phosphorus as added substances isn't bound to protein. Or maybe, it's found as salt and exceptionally absorbable by the intestinal tract (6Trusted Source).

Added substance phosphorus can normally be found in an item's fixing rundown. Be that as it may, nourishment producers are not required to list the accurate amount of added substance phosphorus on the nourishment mark.

While added substance phosphorus substance shifts relying upon the kind of cola, most dim shaded colas are accepted to contain 50–100 mg in a 200-ml serving (7Trusted Source).

Subsequently, colas, particularly those dull in shading, ought to be stayed away from on a renal eating regimen.

Outline

Dull shaded colas ought to be removed from a renal eating regimen since they contain phosphorus in its added substance structure, which is profoundly absorbable by the human body.

2. Avocados

Avocados are regularly touted for their numerous nutritious characteristics, including their heart-solid fats, fiber and cell reinforcements.

While avocados are generally a solid expansion to the eating regimen, people with kidney ailment may need to keep away from them.

This is on the grounds that avocados are an extremely rich source of potassium. One cup (150 grams) of avocado gives an incredible 727 mg of potassium (8).

That is twofold the amount of potassium than a medium banana gives.

Along these lines, avocados, including guacamole, ought to be kept away from on a renal eating regimen, particularly in the event that you have been advised to watch your potassium consumption.

Synopsis

Avocados ought to be dodged on a renal eating regimen because of their high potassium content. One cup of avocado gives almost 37% of the 2,000 mg potassium limitation.

3. Canned Foods

Canned nourishments, for example, soups, vegetables and beans, are regularly obtained as a result of their ease and comfort.

Be that as it may, most canned nourishments contain high amounts of sodium, as salt is added as an additive to expand its timeframe of realistic usability (9Trusted Source).

Due to the amount of sodium found in canned products, it's frequently prescribed that individuals with kidney ailment maintain a strategic distance from or limit their utilization.

Picking lower-sodium assortments or those marked "no salt included" is regularly best.

Moreover, depleting and flushing canned nourishments, for example, canned beans and fish, can diminish the sodium content by 33–80%, contingent upon the item (10Trusted Source).

Synopsis

Canned nourishments are regularly high in sodium. Abstaining from, controlling or purchasing low-sodium assortments is likely best to decrease your general sodium utilization.

## 4. Entire Wheat Bread

Picking the correct bread can be hard for people with kidney infection.

Regularly for healthy people, whole wheat bread is typically prescribed over refined, white flour bread.

Whole wheat bread might be an increasingly nutritious decision, generally because of its higher fiber content. Be that as it may, white bread is generally suggested over whole wheat assortments for people with kidney sickness.

This is a result of its phosphorus and potassium content. The more wheat and whole grains in the bread, the higher the phosphorus and potassium substance.

For instance, a 1-ounce (30-gram) serving of entire wheat bread contains around 57 mg of phosphorus and 69 mg of potassium. In examination, white bread contains just 28 mg of both phosphorus and potassium.

Note that most bread and bread items, paying little respect to being white or entire wheat, additionally contain moderately high amounts of sodium.

It's ideal to think about nourishment marks of different kinds of bread, pick a lower-sodium alternative, if conceivable, and screen your bit sizes.

White bread is normally prescribed over whole wheat bread on a renal eating regimen because of its lower phosphorus and potassium levels. All bread contains sodium, so it's ideal to analyze nourishment marks and pick a lower-sodium assortment.

## 5. Dark colored Rice

Like wheat bread, dark colored rice is an entire grain that has a higher potassium and phosphorus content than its white rice partner.

One cup of cooked dark colored rice contains 150 mg of phosphorus and 154 mg of potassium, while one cup of cooked white rice contains just 69 mg of phosphorus and 54 mg of potassium.

You might have the option to fit dark colored rice into a renal eating regimen, however, if the segment is controlled and offset with different nourishments to avoid extreme everyday admission of potassium and phosphorus.

Bulgur, buckwheat, pearled grain and couscous are nutritious, lower-phosphorus grains that can make a decent substitute for darker rice.

### Rundown

Darker rice has a high substance of phosphorus and potassium and will probably should be parcel controlled or restricted on a renal eating regimen. White rice, bulgur, buckwheat and couscous are for the most part great options.

## 6. Bananas

Bananas are known for their high potassium content.

While they're normally low in sodium, one medium banana gives 422 mg of potassium (16).

It might be hard to keep your everyday potassium admission to 2,000 mg if a banana is a day by day staple.

Tragically, numerous other tropical natural products have high potassium substance too.

In any case, pineapples contain significantly less potassium than other tropical foods grown from the ground be a progressively appropriate, yet delicious, elective.

Synopsis

Bananas are a rich source of potassium and may should be restricted on a renal eating regimen. Pineapple is a kidney-accommodating natural product, as it contains significantly less potassium than certain other tropical organic products.

7. Dairy

Dairy items are rich in different nutrients and supplements.

They're additionally a characteristic source of phosphorus, potassium and a decent wellspring of protein.

For instance, 1 cup (8 liquid ounces) of entire milk gives 222 mg of phosphorus and 349 mg of potassium.

However, devouring a lot of dairy, related to different phosphorus-rich nourishments, can be hindering to bone wellbeing in those with kidney illness.

This may sound astounding, as milk and dairy are regularly suggested for solid bones and muscle wellbeing.

Nonetheless, when the kidneys are harmed, an excessive amount of phosphorus utilization can cause a development of phosphorus in the blood. This can make your bones meager and frail after some time and increment the danger of bone breakage or crack (19Trusted Source).

Dairy items are additionally high in protein. One cup (8 liquid ounces) of entire milk gives around 8 grams of protein.

It might be critical to constrain dairy admission to dodge the development of protein waste in the blood.

Dairy choices like unenriched rice milk and almond milk are a lot of lower in potassium, phosphorus and protein than cow's milk, making them a decent substitute for milk while on a renal eating routine.

# Chapter 3

## Dairy food items: impact on renal diet
Rundown

Dairy items contain high amounts of phosphorus, potassium and protein and ought to be restricted to a renal eating regimen. In spite of milk's high calcium content, its phosphorus substance may debilitate bones in those with kidney infection.

Oranges and Orange Juice

While oranges and squeezed orange are seemingly most notable for their nutrient C substance, they are likewise rich sources of potassium.

One huge orange (184 grams) gives 333 mg of potassium. In addition, there are 473 mg of potassium in one cup (8 liquid ounces) of squeezed orange.

Given their potassium substance, oranges and squeezed orange likely should be kept away from or constrained on a renal eating routine.

Grapes, apples and cranberries, just as their separate juices, are altogether great substitutes for oranges and squeezed orange, as they have lower potassium substance.

Synopsis

Oranges are high in potassium and ought to be restricted on a renal eating regimen. Use grapes, apples, cranberries or their juices.

## 9. Prepared Meats

Prepared meats have for quite some time been related with incessant infections and are commonly viewed as undesirable because of their substance of additives. Prepared meats will be meats that have been salted, dried, relieved or canned. A few models incorporate franks, bacon, pepperoni, jerky and wiener.

Prepared meats ordinarily contain a lot of salt, for the most part to improve taste and safeguard season.

Accordingly, it might be hard to keep your everyday sodium admission to under 2,000 mg whenever handled meats are bounteous in your eating routine.

Moreover, handled meats are high in protein.

On the off chance that you have been advised to screen your protein admission, it's imperative to constrain handled meats consequently too.

Synopsis

Prepared meats are high in salt and protein and ought to be expended with some restraint on a renal eating routine.

## 10. Pickles, Olives and Relish

Pickles, handled olives and relish are generally instances of relieved or cured nourishments.

Normally, a lot of salt are included during the restoring or pickling process.

For instance, one pickle lance can contain in excess of 300 mg of sodium. In like manner, there are 244 mg of sodium in 2 tablespoons of sweet pickle relish (26, 27).

Handled olives likewise will in general be salty in light of the fact that they are relieved and aged to taste less severe. Five green cured olives give around 195 mg of sodium, which is a noteworthy bit of the day by day sum in just a little serving (28).

Numerous markets stock decreased sodium assortments of pickles, olives and relish, which contain less sodium than the conventional assortments.

In any case, even decreased sodium alternatives can in any case be high in sodium, so you will in any case need to watch your bits.

Synopsis

Pickles, prepared olives and relish are high in sodium and ought to be restricted on a renal eating routine.

11. Apricots

Apricots are plentiful in nutrient C, nutrient An and fiber.

They are additionally high in potassium. One cup of new apricots gives 427 mg of potassium.

Moreover, the potassium substance is considerably progressively moved in dried apricots.

One cup of dried apricots gives more than 1,500 mg of potassium.

This implies only one cup of dried apricots gives 75% of the 2,000 mg low-potassium confinement.

It's ideal to avoid apricots: all dried apricots, on a renal eating regimen.

Rundown

Apricots are a high-potassium nourishment that ought to avoided on a renal eating routine. They offer more than 400 mg for each 1 cup crude and more than 1,500 mg for each 1 cup dried.

12. Potatoes and Sweet Potatoes

Potatoes and sweet potatoes are potassium-rich vegetables.

Only one medium-sized prepared potato (156 g) contains 610 mg of potassium, though one normal heated sweet potato (114 g) contains 541 mg of potassium.

Luckily, some high-potassium nourishments, including potatoes and sweet potatoes, can be splashed or drained to lessen their potassium substance.

Cutting potatoes into little, slender pieces and bubbling them for in any event 10 minutes can lessen the potassium content by about half.

Potatoes that are absorbed an enormous pot of water for at any rate four hours before cooking are demonstrated to have an even lower potassium content than those not splashed before cooking.

This strategy is known as "potassium filtering," or the "twofold cook technique."

Albeit twofold cooking potatoes brings down the potassium content, it's critical to recollect that their potassium substance isn't finished dispensed with by this strategy.

Impressive amounts of potassium can at present be available in twofold cooked potatoes, so it's ideal to practice part control to hold potassium levels under tight restraints.

Synopsis

Potatoes and sweet potatoes are high-potassium vegetables. Bubbling or twofold cooking potatoes can diminish potassium by about half.

13. Tomatoes

Tomatoes are another high-potassium natural product that may not fit the rules of a renal eating regimen.

They can be served crude or stewed and are frequently used to make sauces.

Only one cup of tomato sauce can contain as much as 900 mg of potassium.

Sadly for those on a renal eating routine, tomatoes are ordinarily utilized in numerous dishes.

Picking an option with lower potassium substance depends generally on taste inclination. In any case, swapping tomato sauce for a cooked red pepper sauce can be similarly delectable, all while giving less potassium per serving.

Rundown

Tomatoes are another high-potassium organic product that should almost certainly be constrained on a renal eating routine.

14. Bundled, Instant and Pre-Made Meals

Handled nourishments can be a significant part of sodium in the eating regimen.

Among these nourishments, bundled and pre-made suppers are generally the most vigorously prepared and in this manner contain the most sodium.

Models incorporate solidified pizza, microwaveable suppers and moment noodles.

Keeping sodium admission to 2,000 mg for every day might be troublesome in the event that you are eating exceptionally prepared nourishments all the time.

Not exclusively do intensely prepared nourishments contain a lot of sodium, they are regularly ailing in supplements too.
15. Swiss Chard, Spinach and Beet Greens

Swiss chard, spinach and beet greens are verdant green vegetables that contain high amounts of different supplements and minerals, including potassium.

At the point when served crude, the amount of potassium fluctuates between 140–290 mg for each cup.

While verdant vegetables therapist to a littler serving size when cooked, the potassium substance continues as before.

For instance, a half cup of crude spinach will therapist to around 1 tablespoon when cooked. In this manner, eating a half cup of cooked spinach will contain a higher amount of potassium than a half cup of crude spinach.

Moderate utilization of crude Swiss chard, spinach and beet greens is desirable over cooked greens to maintain a strategic distance from a lot of potassium.

Rundown

Verdant green vegetables like Swiss chard, spinach and beet greens are brimming with potassium, particularly when served cooked. Despite the fact that serving size decreases when cooked, potassium substance continues as before.

16. Dates, Raisins and Prunes

Dates, raisins and prunes are regular dried natural products.

At the point when natural products are dried, the majority of their supplements are concentrated, including potassium.

For instance, one cup of prunes gives 1,274 mg of potassium, which is almost multiple times the amount of potassium found in one cup of its crude partner, plums.

Additionally, only four dates give 668 mg of potassium.

Given the noteworthy amount of potassium found in these normal dried organic products, it's ideal to do without while on a renal eating regimen to guarantee potassium levels stay positive.

Outline

Supplements are concentrated when natural products are dried. Along these lines, the potassium substance of dried natural product, including dates, prunes and raisins, is amazingly high and ought to be avoided on a renal eating routine.

17. Pretzels, Chips and Crackers

Prepared to-eat nibble nourishments like pretzels, chips and wafers will in general be deficient in supplements and moderately high in salt.

Likewise, it's anything but difficult to eat more than the suggested segment size of these nourishments, frequently prompting significantly more prominent salt admission than planned.

In addition, if chips are produced using potatoes, they will contain a lot of potassium too.

Synopsis

Pretzels, chips and wafers are effectively devoured in huge segments and will in general contain high amounts of salt. Furthermore, chips produced using potatoes give a lot of potassium.

**Nugget**

In the event that you have kidney malady, decreasing your potassium, phosphorus and sodium admission can be a significant part of dealing with the sickness.

The high-sodium, high-potassium and high-phosphorus nourishments recorded above are likely best constrained or kept away from.

Dietary confinements and supplement consumption proposals will shift dependent on the seriousness of your kidney harm.

Following a renal eating routine can appear to be overwhelming and somewhat prohibitive now and again. Be that as it may, working with your social insurance supplier and a renal dietitian can enable you to plan a renal eating routine explicit to your individual needs.

# Renal Diet Basics

Eating effectively is significant for kidney wellbeing. Individuals with kidney infection need to screen admissions of sodium, potassium, and phosphorus particularly.

Individuals with kidney illness may need to control a few significant supplements. The accompanying data will enable you to alter your eating routine.

If it's not too much trouble talk about your particular and individual eating regimen needs with your PCP or dietitian.

Sodium

Sodium is a mineral found in salt (sodium chloride), and it is broadly utilized in nourishment readiness. Salt is one of the most generally utilized seasonings, and it sets aside some effort to become acclimated to diminishing the salt in your eating routine. In any case, lessening salt/sodium is a significant apparatus in controlling your kidney infection.

Try not to utilize salt when preparing nourishment.

Try not to put salt on nourishment when you eat.

Figure out how to peruse nourishment marks. Keep away from nourishments that have more than 300mg sodium per serving (or 600mg for a total solidified supper). Stay away from nourishments that have salt in the initial 4 or 5 things in the fixing list.

Try not to eat ham, bacon, hotdog, wieners, lunch meats, chicken fingers or chunks, or ordinary canned soup. Just eat soups that have marks saying the sodium level is diminished – and just eat 1 cup – not the entire can.

Canned vegetables should state "no salt included".

Try not to utilize enhanced salts, for example, garlic salt, onion salt or "prepared" salt. Likewise, avoid legitimate or ocean salt.

Make certain to search for lower salt or "no salt included" choices for your preferred nourishments, for example, nutty spread or box blends.

Try not to buy refrigerated or solidified meats that are bundled "in an answer"; or pre-prepared/seasoned. These things are normally chicken bosoms, pork slashes, pork tenderloin, steaks, or burgers.

Potassium

Potassium is a mineral engaged with how muscles work. At the point when kidneys don't work appropriately, potassium develops in the blood. This can cause changes in how the heart thumps, perhaps in any event, prompting a coronary failure. Potassium is found for the most part in leafy foods; in addition to drain and meats. You should avoid specific types

Potassium-rich nourishments to keep away from:

- *Melons, for example, melon and honeydew (watermelon is alright)*

- *Bananas*

- *Oranges and squeezed orange*

- *Grapefruit juice*

- *Prune juice*

- *Tomatoes, tomato sauce, tomato juice*

- *Dried beans – numerous sorts*

- *Pumpkin*

- *Winter squash*

- *Cooked greens, spinach, kale, collards, Swiss Chard*

Different nourishments to keep away from incorporate grain oats, granola, "salt substitute" or "light" salt, molasses. Potatoes and sweet potatoes need unique taking care of to enable you to eat them in SMALL sums. Strip them, cut them in little cuts or solid shapes and absorb them for a few hours a lot of water.

When you are prepared to cook them, pour the dousing water off and utilize a lot of water in the container. Channel this water before you set them up to eat.

Make certain to eat a wide assortment of products of the soil each day to abstain from getting an excess of potassium.

Phosphorus

Phosphorus is another mineral that can develop in your blood when your kidneys don't work appropriately. At the point when this occurs, calcium can be pulled from your bones and can gather in your skin or veins. Bone illness would then be able to turn into an issue, making you bound to have a bone break.

Dairy nourishments are the significant sources of phosphorus in the eating regimen, so limit milk to 1 cup for every day. On the off chance that you use yogurt or cheddar rather than fluid milk – just a single compartment OR 1 ounce daily!

A few vegetables additionally contain phosphorus. Limit these to 1 cup for each WEEK: dried beans, greens, broccoli, mushrooms, and Brussels grows.

Certain grains should be restricted to 1 serving seven days: grain, wheat oats, cereal, and granola.

White bread is superior to anything entire grain breads or wafers.

Soda pops contain phosphorus so just drink clear ones. Try not to drink Mountain Dew® (any sort), colas, root lagers, Dr. Pepper® (any sort). Likewise, evade Hawaiian Punch®, Fruitworks®, Cool® frosted tea, and Aquafina® tangerine pineapple.

Brew additionally has phosphorus – stay away from various sorts.

Individuals images (3) with traded off kidney capacity must stick to a renal or kidney diet to eliminate the amount of waste in their blood. Wastes in the blood originate from nourishment and fluids that are expended. At the point when kidney capacity is undermined, the kidneys not channel or remove waste appropriately. On the off chance that waste is left in the blood, it can adversely influence a patient's electrolyte levels. Following a kidney diet may likewise help advance kidney work and moderate the occurrence of complete kidney failure.

# Chapter 4

# What phosphorus is and its function in the body system

Phosphorus is a mineral that is basic in bone support and advancement. Phosphorus likewise aids the advancement of connective tissue and organs and helps in muscle development. At the point when nourishment containing phosphorus is devoured and processed, the small digestive organs retain the phosphorus with the goal that it very well may be put away during the bones.

## For what reason should kidney patients screen Phosphorus consumption?

Typical working kidneys can remove additional phosphorus in your blood. At the point when kidney capacity is undermined, the kidneys never again remove high levels of phosphorus. High phosphorus levels can haul calcium out of your bones, making them frail. This likewise prompts perilous calcium stores in the veins, lungs, eyes, and heart.

In what capacity would patients be able to screen their Phosphorus consumption?

Phosphorus can be found in numerous nourishments. Hence, patients with traded off kidney capacity should work with a renal dietitian to help oversee phosphorus levels.

# Tips to help protect phosphorus at levels: Phosphorus-Foods

- *Recognize what nourishments are lower in phosphorus.*

- *Give close consideration to serving size*

- *Eat littler parts of nourishments that are high in protein at suppers and for bites.*

- *Eat crisp foods grown from the ground.*

- *Get some information about utilizing phosphate folios at feast time.*

- *Maintain a strategic distance from bundled nourishments that contain included phosphorus. Search for phosphorus, or for words with "PHOS" on fixing marks.*

- *Keep a nourishment diary*

Protein

Protein isn't an issue for solid kidneys. Regularly, protein is ingested and waste items are made, which thus are sifted by the nephrons of the kidney. At that point, with the assistance of extra renal proteins, the waste transforms into pee. Conversely, harmed kidneys neglect to remove protein waste and it collects in the blood.

The best possible utilization of protein is precarious for Chronic Kidney Disease patients as the sum contrasts with each phase of infection. Protein is basic for tissue upkeep and other substantial jobs, so it is critical to eat the suggested sum for the particular phase of sickness as per your nephrologist or renal dietician.

Liquids

Liquid control is significant for patients in the later phases of Chronic Kidney Disease since typical liquid utilization may cause liquid develop in the body which could end up hazardous. Individuals on dialysis frequently have diminished pee yield, so expanded liquid in the body can put pointless weight on the individual's heart and lungs.

A patient's liquid remittance is determined on an individual basis, contingent upon pee yield and dialysis settings. It is indispensable to pursue your nephrologist's/nutritionist's liquid admission rules.

To control liquid admission, patients should:

- *Not drink more than what your primary care physician orders*

- *Tally all nourishments that will soften at room temperature (Jell-O®, popsicles, and so on.)*

- *Be aware of the amount of liquids utilized in cooking*

There is no explicit "renal eating regimen", just rules to enable you to control the degrees of salts in your circulatory system through what you eat. The eating routine required for renal insufficiency fluctuates with each case, the seriousness of the glitch, in the case of growing is available, regardless of whether you are over-weight, what your blood electrolyte readings are, and whether you are a contender for dialysis or not.

With renal failure, the salts in the circulatory system are totally startled. The point of renal eating regimen rules is to help control the development of waste items and liquid in your blood by putting less weight on your kidneys.

Renal eating regimen rules are worked around blood test outcomes and a typical solid adjusted eating routine. The thought is to restrict the admission of salts that are excessively high. Liquids may likewise be confined if your kidneys can't discharge adequate water. Protein admission is restricted so wastes like urea are kept at any rate.

The salts that usually should be confined are:

Sodium can cause hypertension and liquid maintenance. Most renal eating regimens utilize insignificant salt in cooking, and stipulate, "No additional salts". "Lo-salt" mixes are not reasonable for salt substitution as they have high potassium levels and ought not be utilized. Handled nourishments, frankfurters, sauces, ketchups and many canned food sources ought to be maintained a strategic distance from.

Phosphorus can't be removed by dialysis, so it may turn into an issue. Levels are observed, and monitored by eating regimen and now and again prescription. High phosphorus nourishments incorporate dairy items, beans, peas, brew and cola drinks.

Potassium should possibly be confined if the blood levels are high. Numerous healthy vegetables and organic products contain potassium. High potassium nourishments incorporate apricots, squeezed orange, bananas, avocados, beets, spinach and some more.

Proteins are a fundamental piece of a healthy eating routine, yet should just be eaten in modest quantities. Proteins that ought to be confined, incorporate all meats, fish, eggs and dairy items.

Liquids may be limited if water maintenance is available as summed up expanding or liquid in the lungs. Liquids are regularly carefully controlled for patients on haemodialysis. Liquids incorporate all refreshments, soups, water and squeezes.

Starches are vitality nourishments and ought not be confined except if you are a diabetic or overweight. Finally, it may be prudent to take nutrient and cell reinforcement enhancements to help your insusceptible framework.

Following renal eating routine rules will help decline the remaining task at hand on harmed kidneys and hinder the loss of kidney work. The renal eating regimen rules are expected to help keep kidney sufferers solid and useful by eating to help and increase their treatment. It is essential to get explicit guidance from your primary care physician and dietitian consistently.

Renal eating regimens help those experiencing kidney malady to raise their personal satisfaction and how they feel day by day.

Specific kinds of nourishment can be impeding to infected kidneys, so make a point to have a decent working information of the ailment as well as how it influences your body specifically.

Kidney illness isn't something you need, however there are methods for raising your personal satisfaction high by changing your eating regimen. In truth, renal eating regimens help you deal with your wellbeing and keep your kidney malady diminished.

You have to recall changing your eating regimen won't recuperate everybody except it might have the option to support everybody. This doesn't imply that an eating regimen is a fix for everyone so don't think about this article as therapeutic exhortation rather as to a greater extent a rule.

Your primary care physician can give more counsel than this article, and ought to consistently be advised or told of any adjustment in your condition.

On the off chance that you have kidney issues, renal eating regimens are fundamental to managing your wellbeing and helping you in feeling good. There are cookbooks given to renal weight control plans or you could check with an enrolled dietitian for proposals. In the event that you utilize a Kindle or iPad, you can even view these books in a split second.

Dietitians have experience working with those experiencing kidney issues, and can give some broad do's and don'ts to pursue, for example,

**Direct Potassium consumption** - natural products like strawberries and apples alongside vegetables like cauliflower, cabbage and broccoli are low in Potassium.

**Screen your Phosphorous admission -** Non-dairy half and half, pasta, grains and rice are on the OK list.

**Breaking point Fluid Intake -** forty eight oz. of liquid every day is the prescribed level for renal eating regimens make certain to include the liquid in things like grapes, dessert, oranges, and whatnot.

**Screen your salt admission** - You should check to ensure that you keep your salt admission low-comprehend what you are placing into your body and the outcome it might have.

**Manage your admission of protein** - keep up 5-7 ounces. Using egg substitutes rather than customary eggs is a decent method to keep your protein admission low.

Should you use a dietitian, they can point you unequivocally to what you ought to and ought not devour and why. Monitoring the impact nourishment has on your body is incredible data and can help how you feel on an everyday premise. I might want to state again that this organization isn't an option for restorative proposal. Be that as it may, renal eating regimens have energized numerous sufferers of renal illness to move toward becoming and remain more advantageous.

A Renal eating routine is an eating plan worked out to help individuals experiencing renal maladies to support the viability of treatment by limiting the degrees of waste items in their blood.

The renal eating regimen is intended to cause less additional work or weight on the harmed kidneys as could be allowed, while as yet giving adequate great supplements and vitality that the body needs.

A renal eating regimen pursues a few fundamental rules. The main rule is that it must be a reasonable, healthy and feasible eating regimen, plentiful in filaments, nutrients, characteristic grains, sugars, omega 3 fats and liquids. Proteins ought to be sufficient, however not over the top.

The salts that are probably going to aggregate in the circulatory system, are kept to a base. Blood electrolyte levels are observed routinely and the eating routine balanced as needs be. It is imperative to pursue explicit exhortation from your primary care physician and dietitian.

Day by day protein admission is critical to reconstruct tissues, however ought to be kept to a base. Unnecessary proteins should be separated by the body into starches and nitrates. Nitrates are not utilized by the body and must be discharged through the kidneys.

Starches are a significant wellspring of vitality and ought to be taken in sufficient amounts. Entire grains and grungy types of sugars are the best. Maintain a strategic distance from profoundly refined sugars.

Table salt ought to be confined to cooking as it were. Abundance salt causes liquid maintenance and stresses the kidneys. Salty nourishments, for example, handled meats; wieners, many tinned nourishments and tidbits ought to be stayed away from.

Phosphorus is fundamental for the body to work appropriately, yet dialysis can't expel it, so levels should be observed cautiously and admission ought to be constrained however not disposed of. Nourishments, for example, dairy items, vegetables and darker hued beverages like colas, have high phosphorus substance. Nourishments high in potassium content, for example, dull verdant green vegetables, bananas, apricots and citrus natural products, may likewise should be limited if blood levels rise.

Omega 3 fats are a significant piece of any solid eating routine. Greasy fish is an astounding source. Omega fats are basic for solid body working. Keep away from trans-fats or hydrolyzed fats.

Liquids ought to be satisfactory, yet may should be confined in instances of liquid maintenance.

A healthy renal eating regimen can help hold kidney work for more. The principle contrasts between any healthy eating routine and a renal eating regimen, are the limitations put on protein and table salt admission. Limitations on phosphorus, potassium and liquids may end up vital as manifestations and indications of aggregation become clear.

Figuring the essentials of a diabetic renal eating routine is a significant issue as diabetes is the single greatest reason for renal failure. Numerous individuals experiencing kidney issues are additionally diabetics.

Joining a renal eating regimen with a diabetic eating routine has various difficulties. Searching for a satisfactory eating routine for both kidney failure and diabetes can give off an impression of being constraining to the patient from the outset.

The principle objective for a diabetic eating routine is to keep up solid sugar levels in the blood consistently.

There are fundamentally two different ways of accomplishing this:

By just eating starches with a low GI (glycemic file) since they are separated and retained all the more gradually bringing about an unfaltering arrival of sugar into the circulation system over a more extended timeframe. Low GI nourishments incorporate entire grains, grungy nourishments, and most products of the soil, vegetables, sweet potatoes and nuts. Highly refined and thought starches, similar to white bread, confectionaries, sugars and beverages with included sugar ought to be maintained a strategic distance from. They cause glucose "spikes", since they are quickly retained, and will in general wear out similarly as fast.

Eating little regular dinners (around 6 times each day is commonly acknowledged). Remember that it isn't just what is eaten. However, when it is eaten that keeps the glucose levels increasingly consistent. Try not to go significant stretches without eating, and don't eat tremendous suppers or skip dinners.

The renal eating routine then again attempts to reduce weight on the kidneys by decreasing waste items in the circulation system:

By restricting every day protein admission. Overabundance proteins eaten must be separated into sugars and nitrites. The nitrites as urea are disposed of in the pee. This causes superfluous work for effectively harmed kidneys.

Restricting table salt to maintain a strategic distance from water maintenance. Salt substitutions ought not to be utilized as they contain potassium.

The conceivable need to diminish different salts, for example, potassium and phosphates. These are checked by incessant blood tests and just should be restricted on the guidance of your primary care physician. Nourishments with high potassium substance include: apricots avocado, banana, melon, kiwi, citrus natural products, papaya, pears, peaches, prunes and watermelon. A few nourishments with high phosphorus substance are vegetables, dairy, dried vegetables, shellfish, organ meats.

# Diabetic Renal Diet:

Utmost protein admission to roughly 8 oz, or two moderate servings, a day

Eat just low GI sugars

Limit salt, to cooking as it were.

Utmost nourishments with high phosphorus and potassium substance. Follow your doctor's recommendation on this consistently.

Eat little continuous suppers. When you get up toward the beginning of the day, eat your first feast. Eat at 2-3 hourly interims all through the day, taking your last dinner at sleep time.

Tips:

Arranging menus for seven days one after another will enable you to fluctuate your nourishment more.

Plan your day by day nourishment admission so it is spread for the duration of the day

When dishing up nourishment for your primary dinner, fill a large portion of the plate with vegetables or servings of mixed greens, at that point the other half similarly with starches and protein.

Rather than salt, include enhance by utilizing new herbs, non-salt flavors, onions, garlic, a little lemon squeeze or seasoned oils.

For littler dinners eat entire grain oat, saltines or bread, organic product, a glass of skim milk, nuts, yogurt, a little cabin cheddar and a lot of plates of mixed greens.

A diabetic renal diet can be an exceptionally incredible guide in controlling both renal failure and diabetes. It is well advantageous arranging your eating and adhering to your diet. You will feel much improved and be more advantageous for it.

The kidney diet frequently alluded to as the renal diet is intended for individuals with kidney infection. More than 31 million individuals here in the US have kidney sickness and the numbers are expanding. Restorative experts, for example, specialists and emergency clinics working with kidney illness patients built up this unique eating plan with the therapeutic science network and depends on logical research. There is no single kidney diet as each arrangement is explicit to every individual. This requires cautious research and checking so as to structure the right arrangement for every patient needs. The patient needs to work with a renal dietitian to get the correct eating intend to accommodate their dietary necessities. This depends on data, for example, age, movement, on the off chance that they are on dialysis and the level of kidney failure. There are severe rules to control the amount of protein, liquids, phosphorous, potassium and sodium that are devoured, and this helps the kidneys.

Protein is a component that ought to be observed. Protein is expected to fix, keep up and construct muscles, organs and organs. At the point when protein is utilized by the body, it makes urea. Urea is a waste item that is separated from the body in pee by the kidneys. At the point when the kidneys are not working appropriately, urea can develop and cause different genuine diseases. Controlling the sum and sort of protein devoured is important to expand the wellbeing of the kidneys.

Liquids both the sort and the sum can be a significant concern contingent on how much kidney work there is.

Phosphorus and potassium are two different minerals that are found in high sums in various nourishments, for example, organic products, vegetables, nuts, colas and dairy food sources. These minerals are likewise vital for real capacities. The kidneys' errand is to manage the amount of these minerals that are in the body. Having an excess of phosphorus can cause bone misfortune and a lot of potassium can antagonistically influence the heart. Most salt substitutes are made of potassium chloride and are not permitted on most kidney diets. Many low sodium items are presently being made with potassium chloride. You should focus on this to help stay away from a lot of potassium in your diet.

Sodium is imperative to numerous real capacities and can be found in bounty in our nourishments, particularly prepared nourishment, cheap food and café nourishment. One significant capacity that sodium controls the amount of liquid in the body. With a significant level of sodium in the body, thirst is expanded and liquids development. The kidneys help to keep the amount of sodium in the body at the right levels. A lot of sodium admission can put unneeded weight on the kidneys. An excess of sodium has been demonstrated and connected to expanding circulatory strain. Controlling pulse is vital to support the kidneys and keep further harm from kidney illness.

Just quit adding salt to your nourishment at the table or while cooking will help to fundamentally diminish sodium admission. Numerous individuals add salt to their nourishment at the table without really thinking, and just by evacuating the salt shakers can help wipe out that propensity. Try not to cook with salt. Use herbs and flavors. It is additionally critical to avoid salty nourishments like potato chips, salted popcorn, prepared cheddar, and bacon, ham or some other restored meats. Frequently canned, solidified, and handled nourishments are stacked with sodium. It is critical to check the elements of these nourishments for their sodium content. Canned soups are one of those nourishments that can have a colossal amount of sodium. There are presently numerous brands with lower sodium forms. Know these may at present be genuinely high in sodium particularly for kidney patients and might be made with potassium chloride rather than salt.

With such huge numbers of individuals depending on salt to add flavor to nourishment, it is brilliant to find a substitution for it. Many pick normal salt substitutes like crisp lemon juice, or vinegar. They may locate a particular herb or zest like dark pepper, as a flavor they like and use it to include season rather than salt. There are various salt free seasonings without potassium chloride accessible that will securely make progressively delightful low sodium dinners while following the kidney diet.

End stage renal malady (ESRD) happens when incessant kidney infection exacerbates to the time when kidney capacity is under 10% of ordinary. The kidneys neglect to work at a level required for everyday life. Kidneys fundamental capacity is to expel wastes and abundance of water from the body, which gets collected in renal failure prompting harmfulness. The treatment incorporates kidney transplant or dialysis with dietary administration.

ESRD consistently pursues a constant kidney infection; the most widely recognized reason is diabetes and hypertension. Different causes are -

1. Infections influencing supply routes coming to or leaving the kidneys.

2. Innate variations from the norm of kidneys

3. Polycystic kidney sickness

4. A lot of maltreatment of torment meds or different medications

5. Harmful synthetic substances

6. Immune system issue like foundational lupus erythematosus (SLE), scleroderma

7. Damage

8. Glomerulonephritis

9. Kidney stones and optional diseases

10. Reflux nephropathy

11. Different other kidney maladies

Side effects incorporate -

1. General sick inclination and exhaustion

2. Pruritis (tingling) and dry skin

3. Weight reduction without exertion

4. Migraine

5. Loss of craving

6. Queasiness and regurgitating

7. Growing

8. Bone torments

9. Terrible breath

10. Unusually dull skin

11. Changes in nails

12. Draining effectively - wounds, nosebleed, blood in stool

13. Ineptitude

14. Eager leg disorder

15. Restlessness

16. Unreasonable thirst

17. Successive hiccups

18. Amenorrhea

19. Lazy and befuddled state

20. Can't focus or think unmistakably

21. Deadness in various pieces of the body

22. Spasms or jerking of muscles.

23. Irregular wellbeing and lung sounds

24. Decreased or no pee creation

# Chapter 5

# Body framework and liquid in the body system

ESRD prompts development of waste items and liquid in the body, which influences most body frameworks and capacities, including, circulatory strain control, red platelet creation, electrolyte balance, nutrient D and calcium levels and subsequently bone wellbeing. Consequently the patient on dialysis needs to experience different tests regularly to deal with the condition -

1. Sodium

2. Potassium

3. Phosphorus

4. Calcium

5. Magnesium

6. Egg whites

7. Cholesterol

8. Electrolyte

9. Complete blood tally (CBC)

10. Erythropoietin

11. Parathyroid hormone (PTH)

12. Bone thickness test

Treatment and the board -

The executives and treatment of ESRD incorporates kidney transplant or dialysis and dietary administration, it is basic for the patient to know and comprehend everything about the treatment particularly about dialysis and its sorts.

Why dialysis - dialysis removes and keep up waste items, liquid and the electrolyte balance in the body. An extraordinary diet is significant as dialysis alone doesn't viably expel all the waste items. What's more, dietary administration additionally limits the amount of waste development and to keep up the liquid, electrolyte and mineral equalization in the body between the dialysis.

One needs to do bunches of changes in their diet -

ESRD patients need high protein, low sodium, potassium and phosphorus diet and a limited liquid admission. Let's think about each in little subtleties:

Liquid -

Pee output drops during kidney failure. Most dialysis patients pee almost no or not in any way, and subsequently liquid limitation between medications is significant. Without pee, liquid will develop in the body and cause overabundance liquid in the heart, lungs, and lower legs.

Your nutritionist will figure the everyday required level of liquid based on -

• The level of pee yield in 24 hours

• The amount of weight gain between the dialysis treatments

• Amount of liquid maintenance

• Levels of dietary sodium

• Whether you are experiencing congestive cardiovascular breakdown.

Tips -

• Avoid or limit eating nourishment with a lot of water like - soups, harden o, popsicles, frozen yogurts, grapes, melons, palm organic product, coconut water, lettuce, tomatoes and celery.

• Use littler glasses.

• Take tastes of water

• Minimize sodium consumption. Stay away from salty nourishment

• Freeze squeezes in an ice plate and suck them to limit thirst (do include these ice solid shapes in your everyday liquid admission)

• Avoid getting excessively blistering, going out in sun.

Sodium balance -

As said above ESRD patient need to maintain a strategic distance from high sodium diet. Hypertension in ESRD is generally because of positive sodium equalization and volume development (aggregation of a lot of liquid in the body). ESRD patients on dialysis can adequately treat or control hypertension without antihypertensive medications just by having a low sodium diet (2 g/day). Likewise low sodium diet will make you feel less parched and in this way help abstain from swallowing additional liquids.

Tips -

• Avoid - canned, prepared nourishment, handled smoked meat.

• Avoid nourishment with salt garnish viz - chips, nuts and so on.

• Read marks cautiously - select one that peruses - low sodium, no salt included, sodium free, unsalted.

• Avoid nourishments that rundown salt close to the start of the fixing list.

• Choose nourishment which contains salt under 100 mg for every serving.

• Remove salt shaker from the table.

• Cook nourishment without salt rather use herbs for seasoning.

• Avoid safeguarded nourishments - ketchups, sauces, pickles, popadums

• Do not utilize salt substitutes, they contain potassium. What's more, potassium is likewise limited in kidney ailment.

Potassium balance -

Ordinarily a high potassium diet is prescribed to control hypertension and along these lines limit the danger of stroke and cardiovascular breakdown, yet if there should arise an occurrence of ESRD, they can't endure high potassium diet as they can't discharge potassium from their body. High potassium levels in blood will prompt perilous hyperkalemia initiated arrhythmia.

Tips -

• Avoid organic products high in potassium - banana, musk melons, melons, kiwis, honeydew, prunes, nectarines, coconut water, tomatoes, avocado, oranges and squeezed orange, raisins and dried natural products.

• Have organic products like - peaches, grapes, pears, fruits, apples, berries, pineapple, plums, tangerines and watermelon.

• Avoid vegetables high in potassium - spinach, pumpkin, winter squash, sweet potato, potatoes, and asparagus.

• Choose vegetables like - broccoli, cabbage, carrots, cauliflower, celery, cucumber, eggplant (aubergine/brinjal), green and waxed beans, lettuce, onion, peppers, watercress, zucchini and yellow squash.

• Avoid vegetables, milk and wheat grain.

• Limit admission of potassium up to 2 gm for every day.

Iron -

Patients with ESRD will likewise require additional iron.

Tip -

• Consume nourishment high in iron levels - Lima and kidney beans, beet root, green verdant vegetables (maintain a strategic distance from spinach), finger millet, chicken, liver, pork.

• Eat iron braced grains

• Take iron enhancements as prompted by your doctor or dietician.

# Calcium and phosphorus

In ESRD, phosphorous levels are high as it can't be discharged from our body. Indeed, even in beginning periods of renal malady, phosphorus levels can turn out to be excessively high. High phosphorus levels will prompt tingling, vascular calcifications, optional hyperparathyroidism and low calcium levels. In this manner the calcium kept during the bones is spent prompting osteoporosis. Thus a phosphate limited diet is prescribed.

Tips -

• Limit admission of dairy nourishments - milk, yogurt and cheddar.

• Can expend dairy items like - margarine, spread, cream cheddar, full fat cream, brie cheddar, and sherbet as they are low in phosphorus.

• Consult your dietician and take calcium and nutrient D supplement, helps control calcium phosphate levels.

• Avoid caned prepared nourishment.

On the off chance that phosphorus levels are not made do with diet, your doctor may endorse you phosphorus covers.

# Weight Management

ESRD patients' lose weight with no explanation, in this way their weight should be checked and dealt with appropriate adjusted diet. ESRD patients' normal calorie admission diminishes to lower than 30-35 kcal/kg/day prompting hunger. To avoid lack of healthy sustenance related dreariness and mortality, ESRD patients on dialysis need to experience an occasional nourishment screening and tests, contrasting initials body weight and regular and perfect body weight, dietary surveys, and nourishment journal evaluation.
Protein -

You should be befuddled when I state that ESRD patients need high protein, as most realized certainty is patients with renal illnesses should restrict their protein consumption. Valid as when protein separates in our body urea is shaped this can't be discharged in pee and is lethal when it develops in the circulation system. This controlled protein diet is done until patient is put on dialysis. As protein misfortunes are higher in patients experiencing dialysis, they have to expend a high protein diet. Prescribed dietary protein in hemodialysis patients is 1.2 g/kg body weight/day and 1.2-1.3 g/kg body weight/day for patients on peritoneal dialysis. On the off chance that dietary protein - calorie admission isn't sufficient, patients should take dietary enhancements under the direction of a nutritionist, and whenever required they ought to be cylinder feed or parenteral nourishment ought to be given.

Tips -

• Eat top notch protein - fish, pork, eggs, kidney beans, Bengal gram, and soy for each dinner.

• Add egg white or egg white powder or protein powder to your eating regimen.

Sugars -

On the off chance that you are overweight and have diabetes, at that point you need to confine your starch consumption, in any case in the event that you are getting in shape you have to take high sugar diet. As starches are great wellspring of vitality. Your doctor or dietician will prescribe the quantity of carbs required in your eating regimen.

Tips -

• Include - organic products, vegetables, breads and grains, as they are high in fiber, minerals, nutrients and a decent wellspring of vitality.

• If you are prompted a fatty eating routine, devour - hard confections, sugar, nectar, jam, pies, cakes, treats.

• Avoid sweets produced using dairy, chocolate, nuts and bananas.

Fats -

ESRD patients on dialysis are prescribed to restrict admission of immersed fats and cholesterol as they are at high danger of creating coronary supply route sickness. They for the most part have high triglyceride levels, high LDL (low thickness lipoproteins) and low HDL (high thickness lipoproteins). In spite of the fact that you are prescribed to eat a fatty eating routine, you have to keep away from nourishments that raise your triglycerides and cholesterol levels

Tips -

• Include nourishments that are high in monounsaturated and polyunsaturated fats and little of soaked fats. Like - sesame seed oil, flaxseeds, olive oil, and cotton seed oil.

• Avoid canola oil, coconut oil, fats, poultry and chicken with skin.

Micronutrients -

ESRDS patients are prescribed to have a low-fat eating regimen and limited liquid intake. Along these lines numerous patients need to take a nutrient enhancement as fat dissolvable (A, D, E and K) nutrients and water solvent nutrients can't be ingested enough structure the eating regimen and water solvent nutrients are likewise lost during dialysis treatment. For the most part these nutrients are given through vein during the dialysis treatment.

To deal with all the above supplements in the correct amount to suit your needs isn't a simple errand and it is impossible to claim your own. Don't SELF DIET it can hazard your wellbeing. This article is for your data and learning. Counsel a nutritionist who can structure an eating regimen fit for your unique needs. Continuously take your family along to comprehend your dietary needs so they can enable you to pursue your eating routine. In the event that you pursue appropriate eating regimen and physical action as suggested by your doctor and your nutritionist will enable you to feel better and lead a generally solid existence with the ESRD.

Renal diabetes happens because of a low-sugar level in the kidneys. A patient with renal diabetes has ordinary blood glucose levels, however the kidney neglects to reabsorb the typical amount of glucose over into the blood. The high level of glucose is discharged into the circulation system. Renal diabetic cookbooks give plans that take into account the particular healthful needs of these patients.

A renal diabetic cookbook contains an abundance of nourishing data for renal diabetics. Most diabetics complain about the absence of assortment in their menus. Renal diabetic cookbooks help take care of this issue by giving a wide assortment of plans extending from stuffed, heated, steamed, seared, grilled and microwave nourishment.

As a rule, the plans in a renal diabetic cookbook are high in fiber and low in cholesterol, salt, sugar and soaked fat. These books likewise incorporate dietary and cooking style tips that are useful for patients. A portion of these books have areas on arranging unique dinners, for example, canning and solidifying nourishment, and some incorporate the most recent nourishment trade records from the American Dietetic Association and American Diabetes Association. The plans in a renal diabetic cookbook list the dietary benefits of different dishes. This is of extraordinary assistance for a patient who must oversee admission of calories as per the recommended dietary diagram.

Writers of renal diabetic cookbooks look into widely before showing inventive plans for dishes that are commonly not considered a diabetic. For example, a few cookbooks contain plans for delectable sweets, for example, cakes, treats, bars, pies, baked goods and puddings. The fixings and readiness style in every one of these dishes are appropriately changed to fit a diabetics needs.

Most diabetic cookbooks incorporate a segment that manages a posting of calories, starch, protein, fat, sodium, potassium and cholesterol that is contained in each dish. Renal diabetics comprehend the significance of controlling phosphorus. Most renal diabetes cookbook writers remember this when creating plans.

Having a healthy existence is significant and that is the primary target of all of us. There are numerous elements that goes into making an individual healthy and solid and nourishment assumes a significant job. We originate from various sorts of social orders and our societies are unique. With regards to our societies and customs, our nourishment propensities are likewise very extraordinary and it fluctuates from individual to individual, locale to area and nation to nation. While there are numerous nourishment propensities, as indicated by certain individuals adhering on to a vegetarian crude eating regimen is considered as a significant piece of what is known as a healthy nourishment. As we have advanced monetarily and innovatively our nourishment propensities have likewise changed altogether.

We have today part into family units and the idea of joint family which was very applicable in some Asian nations is never again commonsense. Today we have families where the two married couples together have progressed toward becoming providers and henceforth, it has now turned into a standard propensity to go in for readymade nourishment or moment nourishment as it is ordinarily known. These nourishments are by and large are handled in nature and in this manner have various additives that are utilized. Moreover there are wealthy in soaked unsaturated fats which lead to individuals putting on weight and creating cholesterol which start building up in the veins. This causes various medical issues like hypertension, respiratory failures, strokes, renal failure, liver issue and so forth. Henceforth, numerous individuals have begun understanding the significance of veggie lover crude eating routine and have begun moving towards it.

Before we can understand the advantages of these crude eating regimens we ought to comprehend what precisely is a veggie lover crude eating routine? This is an eating regimen that basically comprises of crude foods grown from the ground and different sorts of nuts, vegetables, grain items and organic products fall under this classification. Essentially, these nourishment things are not cooked and are eaten crude. The principal prerequisite for turning into an individual who needs to get by on crude eating regimen, you should abstain from eating any meat items, fish, dairy items, eggs and a wide range of fish. This sounds amazingly intriguing yet, in actuality, it could be a moving change to your way of life. These nourishments are very plentiful in nutrients and minerals, however the inquiry that comes in the psyches of numerous individuals is whether they give our body the necessary amounts of proteins. A few vegetables are great wealthy in sugars and consequently this issue can likewise be comprehended. Be that as it may, the issue stays with just proteins. It is hard to discover numerous organic products, vegetables that are wealthy in proteins. In such a circumstance, you may need to go in for soy protein and start contingent upon nourishment things like tofu. In any case, it could be hard to change in accordance with this kind of eating routine example to start with.

Be that as it may, there are some natural preferences with these sorts of veggie lover crude diet. Most importantly they furnish the body with the correct sort of minerals and nutrients which may get lost as a result of the way toward cooking. Furthermore, since the vast majority of the organic products arrive in a predigested stage it doesn't put superfluous strain and weight on the stomach related framework. They are viewed as the perfect healthy nourishment on account of the way that they are not extremely wealthy in immersed unsaturated fats and henceforth the danger of cholesterol building and fat amassing is diminished to right around zero. These sorts of vegetarian crude diet propensities help to keep our body and mind trim and alert and on the off chance that we can tail it on a long haul premise we could evade all issues of heftiness and lead a typical and illness free life.

Anyway, experts are of the view that vegetarian crude diet is hard to support over significant stretch of time as a result of the way that they don't spoil the taste buds enough and the nonappearance of oil as a cooking medium is something that may not intrigue numerous individuals. They likewise have questions whether these sorts of nourishment propensities would have the option to give the correct sort of calcium and different minerals which nourishment things like milk and fish can gave. Be that as it may, there are some elective leafy foods which have these crucial supplements in bounty. This requires a touch of data assembling and could take some time and endeavors. Be that as it may, the truth remains this is in reality a solid nourishment propensity and on the off chance that one does a cautious SWOT investigation they will clearly discover that the advantages far exceed the disservices. The main thing required to prevail in this veggie lover crude diet is a touch of assurance and duty during the underlying stages. When the body gets used to the diet plan, at that point it would be hard for you to move out from this diet.

Supper substitution projects appear to have turned out to be increasingly more mainstream as of late, and this stresses me a lot!

They arrive in a scope of alternatives, including powders, drinks, soups, bars and rolls. A portion of these items can supplant every one of your dinners, while others supplant a couple of suppers for each day, with the third feast being something solid you cook yourself.

Clearly such projects do enable a few people to get in shape. Be that as it may, there are dangers included.

Studies demonstrate that over the long haul, individuals for the most part can't keep up along these lines of eating long haul, and research has likewise demonstrated that individuals on a 400 calorie for every day diet lose no more weight than those on the 800-calorie diet.

Anyway, why try attempting to pursue such perilously unfortunate low calorie diets?

Extremely low calorie diets can prompt various awkward symptoms. These include:

* Dry mouth

* Headache

* Dizziness

* Fatigue and shortcoming

* Cold narrow mindedness

* Dry skin and nails

* Menstrual abnormalities in ladies

* Hair misfortune

* Constipation/looseness of the bowels

* Irritability and disarray

* Inability to think

* Muscle breakdown

* Problems with nerve and muscle work

* Conditions, for example, osteoporosis, paleness, gout, gallstones, clinical gloom, heart issues, renal failure, and liver ailment

It's critical to take note of that the lower your calorie consumption, the more prominent the probability you will encounter a portion of these reactions. This is exceptionally stressing to be sure!

Extremely low calorie plans, for example, feast swap shakes are unfortunate for various reasons, including:

* They don't empower eating genuine nourishment.

* You chance nutrient and mineral lacks.

* They don't show you how to pick solid nourishment or cook healthy suppers.

It is safe to say that you are as yet considering a dinner substitution plan? I would alert that you first look for the guidance of your primary care physician, and visit an enrolled dietitian for a reasonable and safe arrangement.

On the off chance that you've been battle with inspiration to change your diet, maybe a feast substitution plan isn't the solution to your concern, possibly you first need to change what's happening in your mind, before you can start to chip away at your diet.

Adding healthy nourishment to our regular diet has a lot more included medical advantages than expedient weight reduction and building slender muscle. You will locate that many go about as an incredible detoxifier, wellspring of calcium, wellspring of omega-3 unsaturated fats or go about as against malignancy operators making them extraordinary for clean dietary patterns. Executing certain healthy nourishments into your ordinary diet can help you in long haul solid living by giving your body significant supplements. Here are a couple of instances of solid nourishments that numerous individuals will leave behind in the store that merit a subsequent look.

**Cabbage:** This reasonable and humble verdant vegetable offers you a decent wellspring of Vitamin C, potassium, calcium, folic corrosive, and magnesium. This solid nourishment is likewise a decent wellspring of the amino corrosive glutamine which expands the body's capacity to make human development hormone (HGH). Its mitigating properties help with intestinal wellbeing and insusceptible framework guideline. Studies have shown that expanded cabbage admission offers hostile to malignant growth properties by expanding cancer prevention agent safeguard systems. Incorporate it in your solid nourishment diet by adding it to soup, serving of mixed greens, a Chinese dish or steamed!

# Chapter 6

# Fibre and diet nourishment

Wheat Bran: The wholesome advantages of this solid diet nourishment is undisputed. One cup of wheat grain contains 99% of the US prescribed day by day remittance (RDA) of fiber just as 34% of the RDA for iron and 9 grams of protein, making it a famous mass diuretic. It doesn't stop there! Wheat grain additionally is high in magnesium, manganese, niacin, zinc, nutrient B6 and phosphorous. With no sugar, sodium or cholesterol, thinks about have demonstrated it to likewise work as an enemy of malignant growth specialist advancing ladies' wellbeing and gastrointestinal wellbeing. This low fat solid nourishment fixing is extraordinary for adding to biscuits, hotcakes, waffles, rolls, bread and porridge. At the point when finely powdered, this healthy nourishment fixing can be added to smoothies and yogurt.

Greek Yogurt: Superior to the standard yogurt, Greek Yogurt is higher in protein, lower in starches, thicker, creamier and lower in sodium. One cup of standard yogurt has around 12 grams of protein, while Greek yogurt midpoints around 20 grams! This solid diet nourishment offers significant supplements, for example, calcium for solid bones and osteoporosis anticipation. The live organisms found in it reduce the development of unsafe microorganisms. Greek Yogurt is incredible for breakfast or an early in the day nibble just as a base for solid serving of mixed greens dressings, sauces, smoothies and to supplant cream fixings.

Pink Salmon: This fish is low in immersed fat and high in protein. It offers us omega-3 fundamental unsaturated fat, a wellbeing advancing fat basic for human wellbeing as it can't be made by the body. Omega-3 additionally diminishes aggravation of the veins and stomach related framework, decrease odds of malignancy of the colon, prostate and kidneys, add trying to please, skin hair and nails, improve skin surface and help in the development of advantageous microscopic organisms in the colon. Besides being higher in omega-3 unsaturated fats than other warm water fish, it additionally is an incredible wellspring of selenium, magnesium, absorbable proteins (amino acids), niacin, nutrient B12 and nutrient B6. Pink salmon advances appropriate cardio vascular wellbeing, eye care, viable body digestion and muscle and tissue improvement.

**Broccoli:** A nearby relative of cabbage and cauliflower, this green vegetable can be eaten crude or cooked, however the most ideal ways are to steam them or shallow fry them or eat them crude as serving of mixed greens. This is on the grounds that it helps safeguard the supplements, for example, nutrient C, nutrient A, Vitamin E, zinc, potassium and certain amino acids. Did you know these are additionally great enemy of disease operators? The supplements of this healthy nourishment likewise make it a generally excellent detoxifier, fending off issues related with poisons, for example, joint inflammation, stiffness, gout, tingles, bubbles, rashes, renal calculi and solidifying of the skin. It is wealthy in fiber or roughage, making it the best thing to help fix practically all stomach issue by restoring obstruction. A portion of its other medical advantages incorporate solid skin, invulnerability, bone health, pregnancy nourishment, directs hypertension and shields eyes from Macular degeneration, waterfall and fixes harms from UV radiations. Have a go at steaming broccoli, putting it in the blender and making it a puree with light flavoring as a side for your dish.

A way of life that pursues living nourishments, is reliant on one significant rule - presence! Life starts from presence.

The life of our body is the real totality from the lives in our individual cells. Energetic cells make a completely vivacious body. Healthy tissue makes a healthy body.

How would we create healthy tissue? The guideline can be clarified by the "Life and Death Equation", to be specific: "Better Health" compares to "Life In" in addition to "Death Out".

At the end of the day: much better wellbeing is the consequence of putting more life (living sustenance) in to the body and getting demise, harmful trash, out of the whole body.

What is dwelling sustenance? At the end of the day, its effectively absorbable dinners which haven't been killed, that is, cooked. Along these lines we all promoter great dinners filled in just as devoured crude - like sharp dynamic servings of mixed greens just as perfect new foods grown from the ground natural product juices. Sound appealing?

Think about crude hens and crude pigs, total with plumes, hair, bones, and blood? This likely would wind up being unappetizing for us all. However, not as to genuine animals of unfortunate casualty, genuine carnivores, with teeth, paws and modern quality stomach related framework juices. Concerning such potential predators these kinds of unfortunate casualties may comprise live sustenance!

Anyway shouldn't something be said about dairy items - milk: "nature's primary flawless animal nourishment"? Pleasantly, regardless of whether it's sanitized, that is, readied dead; a calf can't suffer it subsequent to handling. Be that as it may, even in the characteristic express, dairy animals' entire milk and mother's milk are very unique, and not the equivalent to one another as calf milk originate from infants! Obviously, one is

175

perfect for little dairy animals and furthermore the other is phenomenal for the little child.

"Truly, yet will each dinner we devour should be perfect? That is an authentic point. The genuine answer is no". I would state to recollect that every single choice we make has its own belongings. Presently, surely the vast majority of us may expend pretty much whatever we need - and not experience any sort of negative outcomes. In any case, on the off chance that we comprehended that creating certain modifications in eating may enable us to live healthy and energetic life - free from prescriptions and tasks, to our 80s and 90s, it would merit taking considering such positive way of life changes?

The real living nourishments program advertisers an assortment of new natural products, vegetables, just as grew seeds - handled in an assortment of explicit ways - consolidated, aged, not appropriately hydrated, or even squeezed - in spite of the fact that not readied. Besides, we all recommend utilizing wheatgrass natural product squeeze, the genuine organic product juice expelled through entire wheat in its garden type, as one of the most intense kinds of purging sustenance on the planet. All animals instinctively search for the real recuperation power related with low herbage, even household pets!

I'm not catching this' meaning to get passing out of the whole body? This suggests we all try to make the body contamination free. Any dead and additionally toxic fixings in the body ought to be found, killed, and dispensed with - immediately.

All things considered, of the considerable number of organs in your body, likely the most significant might be the intestinal tract. We should acknowledge the obvious issues. At the point when the real colon decelerates, we get defiled just as sick, just as not one in our extra organs, particularly the psyche, can work superbly. On the off chance that the intestinal tract quits working absolutely - or even Lord disallow, breaks - we get dead - rapidly. Consider it on the grounds that comparative towards the sewer cylinder out of your home. At the point when which stops up upward - even mostly - you will realize you have a significant issue. Right? Right!

With the goal, that's the reason we advocate colon cleaning, bowel purges, colonic water system. You ask might it be able to be increasingly agreeable. I would state in no way, shape or form. Is it successful inside mitigating medical issues? That would be viewed as a yes. Presently, in all actuality, we all never wish to wind up controlled by bowel purges, there is no swap for satisfactory dietary fiber, however when the undertaking must be done, start "doing it."

One more thing - nobody accepts that their intestinal tract is blocked. As a matter of fact, there are various degrees of being blocked. Think about this: If my wellbeing is unsatisfactory, just as/or I've been expending for the most part cooked (study: obstructing) suppers my reality, it's an excellent wager that my intestinal tract offers watched much better occasions just as my own medical coverage and way of life may genuinely improve on the off chance that I did some interior housekeeping.

It is basic that everybody have protein in their weight control plans for various reasons, including: to advance muscle development and recuperation, tissue development and recuperation and by and large great wellbeing, also vitality. Yet, it is significantly progressively significant that patients accepting renal consideration have the best possible amount of protein in their weight control plans, on the grounds that various sums are required all through the five unique phases of renal illness. For instance, the individuals who are in stage a couple of their infection need less protein than the normal individual, while the patients who are at the last phase of renal failure, arrange five, require more protein in their eating regimens than the normal individual.

# Dietary Sources of Protein

There are numerous delectable dietary sources of protein that can without much of a stretch be consolidated into any eating routine. Obviously, it is fundamental that any eating regimen plan being trailed by a renal consideration patient must be made by a doctor or dietitian and observed all through the phases of renal failure. Numerous nourishments are exceptionally high in protein, for example, beans, and as long as they are a part of the eating regimen, they are fine to eat.

- Poultry, lean red meat and fish are progressively incredible sources of protein and are stacked with other basic nutrients and supplements. A 100 gram serving of lean red meat contains in excess of 30 grams of protein, making it a marvelous choice for those on low-fat weight control plans. Poultry is another incredible decision for a renal consideration diet, with a 100 gram serving of turkey giving in excess of 25 grams of protein. Fish is a phenomenal alternative, and a most loved remain by, the jar of fish, has 26 grams of protein.

- Nuts, seeds and entire grains are great dietary sources of protein and heavenly as well. This is a brilliant alternative for vegans, just as the individuals who are on low-fat, low-carb slims down. Obviously, the individuals who are hypersensitive to nuts should adhere to seeds and grains. Not exclusively can nuts and seeds make marvelous bites, they can likewise be consolidated into numerous extraordinary plans. Remember about hemp seeds, in light of the fact that in addition to the fact that they are stuffed with protein, they are likewise loaded with cell reinforcements, nutrients and different supplements. Grains can likewise be utilized in numerous plans and are additionally great decisions for morning meals. Dark colored rice, which is additionally utilized much of the time as a protein supplement, is perfect for veggie lovers and is extraordinary eaten either alone or added to plans, for example, chicken soup.

- Although foods grown from the ground don't for the most part have a ton of protein, there are some that are perfect for high-protein slims down. Soy beans are very high in protein, and they are extraordinary for veggie lovers. Soy is additionally one of the sources utilized for protein supplements. Other delectable vegetables that ought to be incorporated into a renal consideration diet incorporate broccoli, carrots, beets, cucumber, mushrooms, lettuce, green peppers, tomatoes, cauliflower, watercress and green peas. There are additionally some flavorful natural products that have heaps of protein, including apples, grapes, bananas, oranges, pears, strawberries, tangerines, watermelons and pineapples.

# Protein Supplements as Part of Renal Care Diets

Numerous patients, particularly in the last phases of renal failure, don't get enough protein in their weight control plans. This frequently happens on the grounds that they have lost their desire for specific nourishments, especially protein nourishments, either because of the flavor or surface. At the point when this occurs, it is regularly prescribed that the patients use protein enhancements to guarantee that they are getting the supplements they need. Protein enhancements are produced using a wide range of sources of protein, including whey, casein, rice and soy. There are various kinds of enhancements accessible, and which ones are utilized relies upon the patient and their needs.

**Whey -** Whey is a finished protein, implying that it contains each of the eight of the fundamental amino acids and every one of the 14 of the unnecessary acids. It is a side-effect of the cheddar making process, and not a decent decision for the individuals who are lactose narrow minded or are sensitive to drain and drain items.

**Casein -** Casein is another finished protein and another milk subordinate. Despite the fact that it comes from milk, numerous individuals who are lactose narrow minded can without much of a stretch review casein, which is more slow acting than whey (in spite of the fact that its belongings last more).

**Rice -** Rice is a fantastic decision for any individual who has sensitivities just as veggie lovers. Rice protein is sans gluten, and it is a finished protein.

**Soy -** Soy is another finished protein and one that is amazing for vegans. A few patients have announced having stomach related issues when utilizing soy, and when this occurs, they find that they should change to an alternate kind of protein supplement.

**Fluid Protein Supplements -** Many individuals, particularly those getting restorative treatment, appreciate the instant fluid protein supplements that are accessible (there are likewise fluid enhancements that are made to be blended into different beverages.) These are helpful and simple to drink.

Protein Powders - Powdered protein enhancements are the most flexible types of enhancements. Not exclusively would they be able to be utilized to make some incredible tasting shakes, smoothies and slushes that can be utilized as dinner substitutions, the unflavored powders can be added to pretty much any formula. Numerous individuals use rice protein for cooking, as it has practically no flavor. The seasoned powders are accessible in chocolate, vanilla, berry, fruit juice and that's only the tip of the iceberg. For a speedy and simple dinner substitution smoothie, it is anything but difficult to several scoops of fruit juice or berry protein powder with one cup of juice (any flavor), one cup of solidified berries, one banana and one half cup of ice. This is blended in a blender, and after that can be delighted in as a delectable, nutrient rich, protein-pressed breakfast.

The main phases of kidney malady generally expedite a confinement the amount of protein you are permitted to have. This will change a lot as the illness advances. You will consistently must be cautious about which supplements you get and in what sums when living with kidney sickness, just as the portion of liquids you can have, however you will most likely need to expand your admission of protein. Your nutritionist will know the careful subtleties you have to keep your wellbeing as near ideal as would be prudent. It will be of indispensable significance to pursue your nutritionist's recommendation cautiously once dialysis winds up vital.

The procedure of dialysis exhausts the degree of protein in your body, which can leave you feeling drowsy and ailing in vitality. It can likewise lessen your fit bulk. Low protein additionally debilitates your resistant framework, leaving you inclined to more diseases and more slow recuperating. It likewise prompts edema, or expanding, for the most part in the feet or lower legs. Your body needs protein to advance recuperating and avoid the improvement of paleness.

Broad blood work will be finished by your therapeutic group to guarantee that you have the correct degrees of protein. Together, a specialist, a medical caretaker and a dietician will search for how a lot of egg whites (a kind of protein) is in your blood. Amazingly low degrees of egg whites are connected to lengthier emergency clinic stays and a further decay of wellbeing for dialysis patients.

Dialysis is just vital when a patient arrives at end organize renal sickness, so it isn't strange to feel powerless and have significantly less of a craving. Tastes will regularly change also. Nourishments overwhelming in protein particularly will frequently taste diverse to a dialysis quiet. This is generally with respect to animal-based protein, which means ingesting more plant-based proteins and protein supplements. The proteins that originate from plants are quite often deficient, which means they don't contain the majority of the fundamental amino acids your body needs. A dialysis patient will require protein to be somewhere close to half and 75% of the complete eating routine.

## For what reason is Protein So Necessary: An In-depth Approach

Notwithstanding the reasons referenced above, protein additionally manages each cell and most elements of your body, for example, making the hormones and compounds that guide in absorption, ovulation and rest. The amino acids found in protein are utilized to make new amino acids. Protein likewise increments and reestablishes your fit bulk, encourages you mend all the more rapidly and battles diseases.

Protein invigorates your body to battle kidney illness, which means you ought to have as much as your PCP will permit.

182

The Many Ways to Get Your Protein

Proteins got from animals are viewed as complete - they contain all the basic amino acids. Animal protein doesn't simply mean meat. It very well may be found in eggs (which some call "the ideal protein"), milk and cheddar. In the event that you long for meat, however are attempting to maintain a strategic distance from fat, there are lean decisions in turkey, chicken bosom and fish. At the point when fat isn't a worry, there is a great deal of protein in meat, sheep and pork, however these ought to be eaten sparingly. Plant proteins are likewise a choice. They are fragmented, as expressed above, yet additionally low in fat and calories. In the event that you are concerned on the grounds that you have nourishment sensitivities or may possibly have them, be cautious when adding new nourishments to your eating routine.

It is constantly a smart thought to keep your eating regimen healthy and shifted with a decent determination of nourishments, however you don't have to have conventional nourishment sources to get your protein. Enhancements come in numerous shapes and structures, including protein bars, protein shots, protein powders, puddings and shakes. In the event that you are searching for a lighter taste, something moderately new is protein water. Before you take any protein supplement, in any case, you ought to counsel with your primary care physician to discover where it can fit into your eating routine. A portion of these may not be as bravo as other protein sources. For instance, a few bars can be an incredible method to get your protein, yet some of them have a high fat and sugar content. An excessive amount of sugar can really mess more up than the protein understands, not the least of which is weight gain, something an end organize renal patient ought to particularly dodge.

There are an assortment of protein powders to pick, including egg, rice, soy and whey. Every single one of these has its very own focal points and inconveniences. Out of them four, just whey is certifiably not a total protein source. Protein powders can be blended into various things so they can be eaten, however they must be blended well. Not doing this appropriately will make the powder and the nourishment unpalatable.

There is another choice for protein - the protein supplement shot.

Eating with End Stage Renal Failure

Meat might be an excessive amount to deal with at this stage, so there should be different approaches to get protein. Perhaps you'll discover eggs are still okay. Eggs are an ideal protein, the source which every other protein are judged. There are various approaches to cook eggs, so you shouldn't become weary of them at any point in the near future. It doesn't damage to include enhancements and protein bars if essential.

Different supplements are as yet imperative to maintain a strategic distance from any extra wellbeing challenges. Bothersome skin, for example, is regularly an indication of a lot of some supplement in the circulation system. You will most likely need to get your blood drawn consistently with the goal that a specialist can screen the degrees of supplements in your blood.

Dialysis may leave you feeling worn out and somewhat peevish. A protein supplement shot may give you the pickup you have to endure rest of the day feeling at any rate somewhat more grounded.

Constant renal failure (CRF) is a typical reason for disease in more established felines. Not at all like some different organs, for example, the liver, can't harm to the kidneys be fixed. Indications of renal illness are typically observed once in any event 70-75% of the renal tissue has been irreversibly harmed and, when built up, CRF is commonly a normally dynamic condition. The pace of movement of infection can shift tremendously from feline to feline. There is no remedy for CRF and in individuals with this condition, dialysis treatment pursued by renal transplantation are the fundamental alternatives. Neither of these medicines are right now accessible in the UK, in spite of the fact that it is conceivable to improve the personal satisfaction of influenced felines by utilizing an assortment of therapeutic medications custom fitted as indicated by the person's needs. As of late numerous treatment advances have been made and there are presently more choices accessible to proprietors wishing to think about their felines with CRF. Before talking about these medicines in detail, it is critical to think about what ordinary kidney capacity is and in this way the scope of issues that felines with CRF may have.

In typical felines, the kidneys assume numerous essential jobs which include:

Disposal of waste items, medications and poisons from the body by means of the pee

Guideline of the body's corrosiveness, electrolyte levels (calcium, phosphate, potassium, sodium and chloride) and water balance

Creation of hormones, for example, erythropoietin (required to animate generation of red platelets by the bone marrow) and renin (significant in controlling water and salt equalization)

185

Initiation of nutrient D (significant responsible for blood calcium and phosphate levels)

## Guideline of circulatory strain

Indications of CRF create when 66% to 75% of renal capacity has been lost. Felines with CRF are defenseless against issues including:

Collection of protein breakdown items (counting urea and creatinine which can be estimated in blood tests) which is related with clinical indications of sickness (for example queasiness, regurgitating, loss of craving)

- *Lack of hydration*

- *Acidosis (expanded blood sharpness)*

- *Electrolyte variations from the norm*

- *Weakness (mostly because of absence of generation of erythropoietin)*

- *Hypertension (foundational hypertension)*

CRF felines regularly give vague indications of sick wellbeing, for example, a variable or poor hunger, weight reduction, gloom and affliction. An expanded thirst is seen in around 33% of felines with CRF despite the fact that this clinical sign can likewise be seen with different conditions basic in moderately aged and older felines, for example, hyperthyroidism and diabetes mellitus ('sugar diabetes'). Finding of CRF in this way requires gathering of blood and pee tests for investigation. Most regularly an analysis is made after recognizable proof of azotemia (amassing of the protein breakdown items creatinine and urea in the blood) and loss of pee concentrating capacity (for example the pee is more weaken than it ought to be). Further tests might be required in certain felines to distinguish the reason for the renal illness. For instance ultrasound assessment of the kidneys is normally a clear strategy for recognizable proof of polycystic kidney ailment (PKD).

The executives of felines with CRF includes a scope of medicines customized by the person's needs.

# What is the perfect diet for felines: Associated with kidney

It is entirely expected to endorse explicit dietary treatment since this has been appeared to improve the personal satisfaction and endurance of felines with CRF and may diminish the pace of movement of sickness. Renal diets commonly have confined degrees of excellent protein which reduces the amount of protein breakdown waste items for the debilitated kidneys to discharge. Levels of phosphate are additionally confined since felines with CRF tend to hold high amounts of this in the body which can add to their inclination unwell. Renal diets have expanded amounts of potassium and B nutrients which CRF felines are powerless against losing in their pee and expanded quantities of calories which aides CRF felines with a poor hunger to keep up a typical body weight. Renal diets generally have lower levels of sodium in them which may decrease the danger of hypertension creating.

It is conceivable to get ready home cooked diets for felines with CRF and veterinary plans are accessible for this reason. Most proprietors don't choose for home cooking conventions as this is very tedious and along these lines not a commonsense alternative by and large.

Felines with CRF frequently have a poor hunger and this can be exacerbated by offering extraordinary kidney diets which may not interest the feline. Now and again, the utilization of hunger stimulants, for example, the counter histamine cyproheptadine (exchange name Periactin) or anabolic steroids can be useful in animating a sufficient craving. All the more as of late a few vets have been treating felines with perseveringly poor cravings by putting a sustaining tube into the stomach. Nourishing cylinders can be put into the stomach utilizing endoscopy and are alluded to as PEG tubes when this is done (percutaneous endoscopically set gastrostomy tube). Albeit a sedative and brief time of post-employable hospitalization is required to put the cylinder, once set up these can be utilized for delayed periods to manage nourishment, fluids and prescriptions to the feline.

In what capacity would dehydration be able to be dealt with and counteracted?

Felines with CRF are helpless against getting to be dried out since they can't deliver concentrated pee. Urging felines to drink and keep up ordinary hydration is useful, if conceivable, and sodden diets are likely ideal. Offering enhanced water may urge felines to drink more (for example fish juices) in spite of the fact that it is imperative to not offer salty fluids as these can build the danger of hypertension and different issues creating. Numerous felines with CRF do anyway lean toward the dry kidney diets and it tends to be hard to empower drinking. Lately, one treatment that has gotten a great deal of consideration is organization of liquids under the skin by the feline's proprietor (subcutaneous liquid treatment).

This isn't at present a typical suggestion in the UK albeit numerous USA proprietors of CRF felines are thinking that it's a straightforward and significant procedure for helping their feline. In extreme cases, drying out may require treatment with intravenous liquid treatment (for example feline admitted to a veterinary medical procedure and set on a dribble). Giving extra liquids at home can thusly be useful in anticipating this. What's more, additional medicines, for example, potassium can be added to the liquids. Subcutaneous liquid treatment as a rule includes giving around 150 ml of liquid under the skin two times every week. The procedure is very much endured by most felines and proprietors incorporate one report of a multiyear old feline with CRF that has been overseen for a long time utilizing subcutaneous liquid treatment as a component of the administration convention. In the event that fundamental, the system can be changed to increasingly visit liquid organization. The proprietor will be prepared in how to play out this strategy by a veterinary specialist or medical caretaker - it is significant that the liquid is given accurately in a clean way so diseases don't happen at the site of infusion. A few felines don't endure this strategy thus it may not be appropriate for all felines with CRF.

In what manner can electrolyte issues be dealt with and anticipated?

Electrolytes are salts present in the body which are required for typical cell capacities. The most well-known electrolyte awkward nature in CRF felines include potassium and phosphate. CRF felines are defenseless against losing potassium in their pee which can cause a decrease in the blood potassium levels (hypokalemia). Hypokalemic felines can turn out to be exceptionally powerless and lose their hunger. Albeit renal diets contain expanded amount of potassium in them, a few felines with CRF can in any case grow low blood potassium levels. Extra potassium can be provided to these felines as a powder, tablet or fluid.

CRF felines are defenseless against collecting phosphate which can make them hyperphosphataemic (have high blood phosphate levels). Oral phosphate fasteners are drugs which tie to phosphate present in the diet and utmost what is consumed by the feline's gut. These medications might be required in CRF felines whose blood phosphate levels remain high regardless of dietary treatment or in those felines that won't eat a remedy diet.

In what capacity can foundational hypertension be dealt with and avoided?

(Hypertension) happens in 20 - 30% of felines with CRF and can have genuine outcomes, for example, visual impairment. Checking of circulatory strain is accordingly significant with the goal that hypertension can be distinguished and treated quickly where it happens. Most practices currently have offices to gauge pulse in felines and this is a strategy which is straightforward, torment free and just takes a couple of minutes to perform. In those felines requiring treatment, hostile to hypertensive medications, (for example, oral amlodipine or benazepril) can be endorsed. Most felines need once every day treatment to keep up ordinary pulse.

www.ingramcontent.com/pod-product-compliance
Lightning Source LLC
Chambersburg PA
CBHW062134020426
42335CB00013B/1208